The Palgrave Macmillan Animal Ethics Series

In recent years, there has been a growing interest in the ethics of our treatment of animals. Philosophers have led the way, and now a range of other scholars have followed from historians to social scientists. From being a marginal issue, animals have become an emerging issue in ethics and in multidisciplinary inquiry. This series will explore the challenges that Animal Ethics poses, both conceptually and practically, to traditional understandings of human-animal relations. Specifically, the Series will:

- provide a range of key introductory and advanced texts that map out ethical positions on animals
- publish pioneering work written by new, as well as accomplished, scholars;
- produce texts from a variety of disciplines that are multidisciplinary in character or have multidisciplinary relevance.

More information about this series at
http://www.palgrave.com/gp/series/14421

Rebecca Rose Stanton

The Disneyfication of Animals

palgrave
macmillan

Rebecca Rose Stanton
Northumbria University
Newcastle upon Tyne, UK

The Palgrave Macmillan Animal Ethics Series
ISBN 978-3-030-49315-8 ISBN 978-3-030-49316-5 (eBook)
https://doi.org/10.1007/978-3-030-49316-5

This Palgrave Macmillan imprint is published by the registered company Springer Nature Switzerland AG.
The registered company address is: Gewerbestrasse 11, 6330 Cham, Switzerland

Series Editors' Preface

This is a new book series for a new field of inquiry: Animal Ethics.

In recent years, there has been a growing interest in the ethics of our treatment of animals. Philosophers have led the way, and now a range of other scholars have followed from historians to social scientists. From being a marginal issue, animals have become an emerging issue in ethics and in multidisciplinary inquiry.

In addition, a rethink of the status of animals has been fuelled by a range of scientific investigations which have revealed the complexity of animal sentiency, cognition and awareness. The ethical implications of this new knowledge have yet to be properly evaluated, but it is becoming clear that the old view that animals are mere things, tools, machines or commodities cannot be sustained ethically.

But it is not only philosophy and science that are putting animals on the agenda. Increasingly, in Europe and the United States, animals are becoming a political issue as political parties vie for the "green" and "animal" vote. In turn, political scientists are beginning to look again at the history of political thought in relation to animals, and historians are beginning to revisit the political history of animal protection.

As animals grow as an issue of importance, so there have been more collaborative academic ventures leading to conference volumes, special journal issues, indeed new academic animal journals as well.

Moreover, we have witnessed the growth of academic courses, as well as university posts, in Animal Ethics, Animal Welfare, Animal Rights, Animal Law, Animals and Philosophy, Human-Animal Studies, Critical Animal Studies, Animals and Society, Animals in Literature, Animals and Religion – tangible signs that a new academic discipline is emerging.

"Animal Ethics" is the new term for the academic exploration of the moral status of the non-human – an exploration that explicitly involves a focus on what we owe animals morally, and which also helps us to understand the influences – social, legal, cultural, religious and political – that legitimate animal abuse. This series explores the challenges that Animal Ethics poses, both conceptually and practically, to traditional understandings of human-animal relations.

The series is needed for three reasons: (i) to provide the texts that will service the new university courses on animals; (ii) to support the increasing number of students studying and academics researching in animal related fields, and (iii) because there is currently no book series that is a focus for multidisciplinary research in the field.

Specifically, the series will

- provide a range of key introductory and advanced texts that map out ethical positions on animals;
- publish pioneering work written by new, as well as accomplished, scholars, and
- produce texts from a variety of disciplines that are multidisciplinary in character or have multidisciplinary relevance.

The new Palgrave Macmillan Series on Animal Ethics is the result of a unique partnership between Palgrave Macmillan and the Ferrater Mora Oxford Centre for Animal Ethics. The series is an integral part of the mission of the Centre to put animals on the intellectual agenda by facilitating academic research and publication. The series is also a natural complement to one of the Centre's other major projects, the Journal of Animal Ethics. The Centre is an independent "think tank" for the advancement of progressive thought about animals, and is the first Centre of its kind in the world. It aims to demonstrate rigorous intellectual enquiry and the highest standards of scholarship. It strives to be a world-class centre of academic excellence in its field.

We invite academics to visit the Centre's website www.oxfordanimalethics.com and to contact us with new book proposals for the series.

General Editors
Andrew Linzey and Clair Linzey

Contents

Introduction

This book explores how animal harm and objectification are depicted in the fifty-six Walt Disney Animation Studios (hereafter: WDAS) films from 1937–2016, beginning with *Snow White* and ending with *Moana*. Since 1937, the treatment of non-human animals (hereafter: animals) in the Anglo-American world has changed for both the better and the worse. By August 2016, there were more laws and charities than ever before to protect animals from harm, yet there were also record numbers of animals being routinely mistreated and killed for the production of food. Some of the routine harm and objectification that animals commonly experience are depicted in WDAS films, but other forms are not. This book will demonstrate that whether or not animal harm and objectification are depicted in WDAS films depends upon four factors: the social acceptance of the harm or objectification, the species affected, the number of animals involved, and how visible the harm is to humans (in both film and reality).

Animals populate every WDAS film, and their roles vary greatly. They have been depicted as protagonists, pets, best friends, background characters, and much more. They also commonly appear in objectified forms: as meat, leather, and so forth.[1] Their characterization or objectification within WDAS films depends largely on the species of animal they are based on. For example, as primary characters, rats are always villainous.

[1] Within this text, "objectification" refers to the literal reduction of animal to object. For example, a cow being processed into a hamburger. This book will not use "objectification" to refer to symbolic objectification (such as a live tiger caged in a zoo) unless explicitly stated.

They also commonly exist as minor characters to symbolize a dangerous location, such as a witch's dungeon. In contrast, dogs are usually detailed, heavily-anthropomorphised, individualized, neotenous, pro-social characters that are depicted as loyal, friendly, and undeserving of even minor harm, such as name-calling. To illustrate, in *Lady and the Tramp* (1955), the pet dogs are heavily anthropomorphised, neotenous, and detailed. The narrative repeatedly implies that dogs should be respected and not harmed in any way. Yet in the same film, the villainous non-anthropomorphised rat character is unceremoniously killed by one of the dogs, which is portrayed as a justified action by the dog. Further to this, some species, such as cows, are more frequently depicted in their objectified form (as meat or leather) than in their living form. Yet other commonly-depicted species, such as cats, never appear in an objectified form. Thus, an animal's species very much determines the harm or objectification it experiences in WDAS films, as well as its characterization.

Animals, both living and objectified, pervade WDAS films. However, in most WDAS films that feature animals, or products made from animals, something significant is missing: the processes that transform animals into objects, such as those that occur in slaughterhouses. Additionally, the routine mistreatment animals frequently experience in reality, such as being caged, is rarely depicted by WDAS. When WDAS does depict harm towards animals, it is often romanticized, which is particularly evident with their[2] depictions of animal farming and pet ownership as Chaps. 1 and 4 will demonstrate respectively. However, the fact that WDAS films commonly romanticize animal harm and objectification is unsurprising given that WDAS romanticizes many challenging areas of life. For example, WDAS films often romanticize poverty. To illustrate, *Cinderella* (1950) optimistically depicts the destitute, overworked, and verbally-harassed Cinderella as content with her miserable situation. However, Walt[3] was well documented to be proud of the

[2] "WDAS" is being used as a singular noun in this text. However, the pronouns used to refer to WDAS in this text are they/ their/ themselves and *not* it/itself. This is also true of "Disney", "PETA", and the "AHA".

[3] This book will refer to Walt Disney (the person) as "Walt" rather than "Disney". While people should be referred to by their surname in academic writing, to do so would be confusing with Walt Disney in this book because the main focus is Disney films. In this text, "Disney" will refer only to

romantic nature of his films. For example, in response to criticism that his films were too sweet, he famously said that: "There's enough ugliness and cynicism in this world without me adding to it" (Walt, in: Schickel 2019: 58). This seems to confirm that WDAS's romanticism of complex issues was intentional, at least in the studio's early days.

The scope of this text begins in 1937, with a film that changed animation, film, and Anglo-American culture overnight. *Snow White and the Seven Dwarfs* was an expensive risk that many doubted would succeed (Wasko 2001: 14). However, it was a gamble that paid off handsomely; *Snow White* was a resounding critical and financial success. As a result, it has received much academic attention from film scholars (for example: Inge 2004: 132–42; Kalmakurki 2018: 7–19; Layng 2001: 197–215). Despite this, the film's many animal characters, and the harm or objectification they experience, have not yet been studied in sufficient detail. Yet, there is much to be said about these elements of the film. The opening shot of *Snow White* depicts the angelic Snow White scrubbing steps and singing tunefully to a dole of adoring, slightly-anthropomorphised, white doves. Prince Charming enters the scene soon after with a non-anthropomorphised horse by his side and a large fluffy white feather in his regal blue cap. This moment – the first time that WDAS depicts animals – not only establishes how ubiquitous animals are in WDAS films, but it also captures three very different depictions of animals that will be focused on individually within this book: as anthropomorphised beings that interact with the human characters (the doves), as subservient non-anthropomorphised beings (Prince Charming's horse), and as objects (the white fluffy feather in Prince Charming's hat). However, the main focus of this book is animal harm and objectification, so the feather and Prince Charming's subservient horse is what this text will analyse in detail. Yet the doves are still significant as they present the romantic alternative to animal harm and objectification that is commonplace in WDAS films. As *Snow White* continues, more animal characters and objects appear, and more harm and objectification are evident. To illustrate, the

---

the general Disney company. Similarly, "Roy Disney" (Walt's brother) will be referred to as "Roy". This is consistent with other recent Disney scholarship, such as Davis (2007). All other people will be referred to by their surname.

huntsman who takes Snow White to the forest wears leather clothing, and the dwarfs use a deer to pull their mining cart. Moreover, certain species (such as doves) are clearly associated with pro-social characters and safe situations, yet other species (such as bats, rats, and eagles) are clearly associated with anti-social characters and danger. For example, when Snow White subsequently gets lost in the forest, she is frightened by a cloud of black bats; rats populate the evil stepmother's potion-making dungeon; eagles gleefully follow the stepmother as she falls off a cliff to her death. Additionally, certain species experience socially-acceptable harms, and other species do not. For example, the bird whose feather decorates Prince Charming's hat is never mentioned; therefore, the objectification of this bird is only implied and is thus contextualised as being acceptable. In contrast, the anthropomorphised, neotenous, subservient rabbits that assist Snow White with cleaning and cooking face no harm or objectification at all. As this book will evidence, this discrimination between different species recurs throughout WDAS's outputs. It was not until 2016's *Zootopia*, the second last film included in this text, that these speciesist attitudes were challenged.

Book Structure

Each of the five chapters in this book will explore how a different form of animal harm or objectification have been depicted within WDAS films. The forms of harm or objectification discussed are the ones that have been the most commonly depicted by WDAS. Some common forms of animal harm, such as medical testing, have never been depicted, or even referenced, in any WDAS film. Thus, there is not enough information to warrant a full chapter on these types of harm or objectification. Each chapter will begin by summarizing the literature, history, and theories relevant to that specific area of harm or objectification. Each chapter also contains at least one WDAS film case study relevant to that topic. The specific filmic case studies in each chapter were chosen because they explicitly depict the harm or objectification relevant to that chapter's topic. For example, *Brother Bear* depicts both hunting and fishing, making it an appropriate case study for Chap. 2. Therefore, previously under-studied WDAS works, such as 2004's *Home on the Range*, will be explored in this text, countering the tendency in prior research to focus on WDAS's more commercially-successful films. To illustrate, *Beauty and the Beast* (1991) has received much more academic attention than some other, less financially-successful, WDAS films (for example: Cummins 1995: 22–28; Olson 2013: 448–480).

In order to better understand ideas of animals and animal harm, this text will utilize several theories. Firstly, this text will utilize ideas of speciesism, which is defined as "the unjustified disadvantageous consideration or treatment of those who are not classified as belonging to one or more particular species" (Horta 2010: 244). It is claimed that speciesist attitudes are based on a "socio-zoological scale" of value (Arluke and Sanders 1996). This scale determines how important a species is, or is not, to humans. For example, cats score very highly on this scale, whereas cockroaches score very low. A species rank is determined by the following five criteria: usefulness, relationship to humans, appearance, danger factor, and how demonic the animal is to humans (Arluke and Sanders 1996). The socio-zoological scale is vital to this text and will be used in every chapter to describe the status of WDAS's animal characters alongside speciesism. Secondly, this text will often refer to the "collapse of compassion" effect. It has been repeatedly demonstrated that humans care more about animals when they are presented as named individuals, rather than when they are shown in groups (Payne 2010). Generally, the more victims a tragedy has, the less humans will care, and the less-likely they are to donate their time or money to help solve the situation (Payne 2010; Cameron et al. 2011: 1). This is termed the "collapse of compassion" effect. Thirdly, this text will often reference romanticism, particularly in relation to how animal harm is depicted in cultural representations. The term "romanticism" is said to have several meanings. This book will define "romanticism" by using the definition that is sometimes referred to as a misunderstanding of it, that is, someone who romanticizes the past or present (Ruston 2007). However, this definition is only seen as a misunderstanding when used to refer specifically to the romantic British poets, which is not the case in this book (Ruston 2007).

Chapter 1 will examine depictions of animal food farming, encompassing meat production, dairy farming, farmhouses, farmers, and the various species that usually live on farms in WDAS films. Part I of this chapter will explore the history of animal farming, and the common tropes that are evident in notable cultural representations of it. Part II will document how often farm locations, farm animals, and the products of farming (meat and so forth) have been depicted in WDAS films. Part III will analyse key depictions of farming within WDAS films, concluding that WDAS is complicit in keeping the "happy farm" myth alive. It will also explore the limited ways in which WDAS has depicted characters that consume farm products, such as meat. Finally, Part IV will examine *Home on the Range* (2004), a WDAS film set on a dairy farm that reinforces many misconceptions about the farming industry, the tone of which is shaped by romanticism and comedy. This chapter will conclude by arguing that WDAS's image of animal farming has been consistently unrealistic and saccharine, even though life has evidently become far worse for farm animals during the period in which WDAS has been producing films. This is because over the past one hundred years, farming has become increasingly industrialised and efficient, to the detriment of animal welfare.

Chapter 2 will focus on WDAS's depictions of hunting and fishing. Hunting and fishing are analogous practices; they both involve tracking and (usually) directly killing an animal. However, these practices differ in terms of the species involved, the location of the practice, and the degree to which they are socially accepted. Part I of this chapter will explore the history and current discussions surrounding these two practices. For example, it will question why trophy hunting has become socially-unacceptable, yet fishing is still socially-acceptable. Then, Part II will document the frequency with which these practices have been depicted in WDAS films. Next, Part III will explore how WDAS has portrayed hunting and fishing, paying particular attention to how hunted and fished animals have been depicted, as well as the portrayal of humans who participate in these practices. Finally, Part IV will concentrate on how hunting and fishing were portrayed in 2003's *Brother Bear*. *Brother Bear* was chosen for this chapter's case study because it reinforces the idea that hunting mammals is immoral, but that fishing is socially-acceptable. This chapter will conclude by arguing that the manner in which WDAS has depicted hunting and fishing reflects common speciesist attitudes.

Additionally, WDAS has helped to sustain these speciesist attitudes with their own texts. Since hunting (as a hobby in contemporary Anglo-American culture) is broadly no longer socially-acceptable, it is rarely romanticized in WDAS films. It is only depicted as socially-acceptable when committed by indigenous people or towards villainous animals. This is true both in WDAS films and wider media.

Chapter 3 will examine how WDAS has depicted clothing and other objects made from animals' bodies, such as fur coats, leather books, and feather quills. While the production of fur has become socially-unacceptable in the Anglo-American world, the production of leather, feathers, and so forth, are still widely considered to be socially-acceptable. Part I of this chapter will outline the relevant history surrounding clothing and other objects produced from animals' bodies. It will explore why similar products made from different species have been responded to very differently. It will also illustrate how PETA[4] has campaigned, both successfully and unsuccessfully, against the production of fur, leather, and so forth. Part II will provide data that demonstrates how often these products have been depicted in WDAS films. Then, Part III will delineate how WDAS has depicted fur products, compared to how they have depicted other products made from animals' bodies (such as leather-bound books and feather quills). Finally, Part IV will scrutinise WDAS's most famous film about the ethics of producing clothing from animals: *One Hundred and One Dalmatians* (1961). This chapter will conclude by claiming that WDAS is selective with their criticism of products made from animals' bodies. Comparisons will be drawn to the inconsistencies highlighted in Chaps. 1 and 2 with farming, hunting, and fishing. This is because the social-acceptance of clothing made from animals depends significantly on both the species affected and the demographics of the human consumer, which is also true of farming, hunting, and fishing.

[4] PETA (People for the Ethical Treatment of Animals) claims to be the largest animal welfare charity in the world with 6.5 million members (*PETA* 2019a). They focus their campaigns on the four areas in which they believe animals suffer the most: laboratories, the food industry, the clothing trade, and the entertainment industry (*PETA* 2019a). Because of their broad scope, PETA's campaigns and research will be utilized throughout this book. However, it must be acknowledged that PETA is often criticized for various reasons, some of which will be discussed in the chapters of this text (for example: McWilliams 2012).

Chapter 4 will assess depictions of pets and working animals in WDAS films. These two types of characters are widespread in WDAS films. That prevalence perhaps reflects how central pets and working animals have been in human cultures throughout history. Part I will explore that history, outlining the common ethical objections towards keeping animals as pets and using animals as labourers. Part II will quantify how often pets and working animals have been depicted in WDAS films, documenting the species, scale of anthropomorphism, and purposes that these characters serve. Then, Part III will examine this data, highlighting the types of direct and indirect harm and objectification these animals face in WDAS films. Finally, Part IV will examine *Lady and the Tramp* (1955), a WDAS film that focusses on pet animals and also features various working animals. This chapter will conclude by claiming that direct harm towards non-villainous pets appears to be acknowledged and criticized more than any other type of animal harm in WDAS films. In contrast, working animals tend to face routine physical harm, which is rarely criticized or even acknowledged by WDAS. This chapter will conclude by stating that this disparity reflects wider socially-acceptable speciesist attitudes towards these two types of animals.

Chapter 5 will explore how animals in entertainment have been depicted in WDAS films. This is one of the most-debated and controversial areas of animal welfare. This is evident from the many high-profile campaigns surrounding this issue, several of which will be highlighted and discussed in this chapter. Part I of this chapter will explore the most common objections towards using animals for entertainment. Part II will document the number of times animal performance has been depicted in WDAS films. Part III will begin by outlining the history of zoos and circuses. Then, this section will focus on how WDAS has depicted these locations. This section will employ *Dumbo* (1941) as a case study. Finally, Part IV of this chapter will contextualise the use of animals in the North American (hereafter: American) film industry. It will begin by examining the history of animal actors in American films, and then it will explore how WDAS has depicted animal actors. This section will employ *Bolt* (2008), a CGI film about the ethics of using animals as actors, as a case study. This chapter will conclude by arguing that it has evidently become socially-unacceptable to use animals to produce entertainment. A study of WDAS films and numerous welfare campaigns will demonstrate that this issue has garnered attention because animal performers are higher-order species that are typically individualized.

This text's conclusion will highlight several original contributions to knowledge that have been made apparent from the chapters of this book. First, the conclusion will demonstrate that WDAS films reflect speciesist attitudes. WDAS films repeatedly imply that it is unacceptable for certain species, such as dogs and elephants to be harmed, yet WDAS films also imply that is socially-acceptable to harm other species, such as fish and insects. Second, WDAS has only challenged animal welfare issues that are already socially-unacceptable, or are becoming socially-unacceptable. Moreover, they only question harms that affect small numbers of animals, such as the use of animals in entertainment. Third, WDAS repeatedly romanticizes, humourizes, and minimizes the routine harm and objectification that animals experience during processes that are potentially harmful, such as dairy farming. Fourth, WDAS films can influence how viewers feel towards animal welfare, perhaps more so than even many animal-centred organizations, such as PETA. Fifth, individualization significantly influences how viewers feel towards animals, even when these animals are fictional and animated. Sixth, the amount of harm an animal character experiences, and how much sympathy the narrative offers that animal, depends largely on how anthropomorphised that character is. It is often implied that heavily-anthropomorphised animals should not be harmed. In contrast, non-anthropomorphised animals are often depicted experiencing harm that is portrayed as acceptable. Seventh, since WDAS films rarely feature violence towards animals (which is the most prevalent form of violence globally), WDAS fails to depict scale of harm done to animals in the real world. Animals exist in every WDAS film, yet their most common causes of death (slaughterhouses and so forth) have barely been mentioned. Therefore, in WDAS films, animals are disconnected from the harms they often experience in reality.

WDAS has benefitted from animals in the sense that some of their most memorable films and scenes feature animal characters. Thus, WDAS owes their unique success and global prevalence to their many anthropomorphised neotenous animal characters. However, WDAS has shown little interest in the problems most animals face. For example, during WDAS's history (1937–present), farming has moved increasingly towards industrialised efficiency, and the numbers of animals involved has risen exponentially. Today, animal farming kills more land animals than any other industry. Since WDAS films include numerous images of farms but do not depict the reality of modern farming, they are complicit in propagating misleading images, and consequently the continuation of poor animal treatment. WDAS (and Disney) are not directly responsible for the problems associated with farming; however, given how large and global their audience is, they have the ability to improve public knowledge about contemporary agricultural practices. Additionally, given that WDAS has the attention of many children, they have a responsibility to consider the attitudes embedded within their narratives. While WDAS continues to negate the realities of contemporary industrialised farming, they are suggesting that there are few problems associated with it. These points will be examined in detail in the first chapter of this text: animal farming in WDAS films.

1

WDAS's Problematic Portrayal of Food Farming

If you're gonna kill the cow, I don't wanna hear the rest of the story
– Mortimer Snerd, *Fun and Fancy Free* (*1947*)

The quote above is taken from "Mickey and the Beanstalk", the second half of WDAS's *Fun and Fancy Free* (1947). This short film opens with images of fertile fields that are inhabited by happy, free-range, farm animals living comfortably in small numbers. However, the fields become barren overnight after an antagonistic giant steals the town's magic harp. As a result, three humanoid farmers – Mickey Mouse, Goofy, and Donald Duck – become starving and destitute. All they have left is their farm and cow. Upon hearing this, the little girl listening to the story optimistically exclaims: "At least they had milk".[1] It is then apparent that even though the three farmers are starving, they have not eaten their dairy cow. Instead, the farmers share a vegan meal: a tiny slice of bread and a single bean. However, after going mad with hunger, Donald Duck tries to kill their

[1] *Fun and Fancy Free* features two short films, "Bongo" and "Mickey and the Beanstalk". "Mickey and the Beanstalk" is narrated by notable ventriloquist Edgar Bergen who tells the story in live-action to a young girl with his ventriloquist dummies, which is segmented between the animation.

R. R. Stanton, *The Disneyfication of Animals*, The Palgrave Macmillan Animal Ethics Series, https://doi.org/10.1007/978-3-030-49316-5_1

cow with an axe. He is stopped by Mickey and Goofy, who are both horrified by Donald's murderous intentions. Upon hearing that Donald planned to kill their cow, the little girl announces that this is terrible given that the cow was their "best friend". One of the ventriloquist's puppets then suggests several gruesome and cartoonishly-dramatic ways that the farmers could kill their cow, such as by pushing her off a cliff whilst she sleeps. This is when Mortimer Snerd states: "If you're gonna kill the cow, I don't wanna hear the rest of the story". Of course, the dairy cow is not killed or harmed in any way. Therefore, "Mickey and the Beanstalk" depicts a farm cow as a character worthy of a life without harm. It also implies that farmers do not harm animals, even in desperate circumstances. Both of these points are unrealistic given the harsh reality of agriculture both today, and when *Fun and Fancy Free* was produced and set.

This first chapter will explore WDAS's portrayal of animal farming. This will include analyses of meat production, dairy farming, farmhouses, farmers, and the various animals that usually live on farms in WDAS films. These concepts will be studied alongside theories of romanticism and speciesism, two techniques often used to justify, attenuate, and hide the harsh realities of modern animal farming. This chapter will also note the influence that the "collapse of compassion" has upon farm animals. Part I of this chapter will explore the history of animal farming, and the common and notable cultural representations of it. Part II will list how often farm locations, farm animals, and the products of farming (such as meat) have been depicted in WDAS films. Part III will analyse farming in WDAS films, concluding that WDAS is complicit in keeping the "happy farm" myth alive. It will also look at the limited way in which WDAS has depicted characters that eat farm products, such as meat. Finally, Part IV will examine *Home on the Range* (2004), a WDAS film set on a dairy farm. This film supports many of the misconceptions about the farming industry that are commonplace in cultural representations, the tone of which is shaped by romanticism and comedy. This chapter will conclude by arguing that WDAS's portrayal of farming has been consistently unrealistic and saccharine, even though over the past one hundred years, industrialisation and striving for efficiency (under capitalism) have been detrimental to animal welfare.[2]

Part I: The History and Romance of Animal Farming

The exact number of animals reared and slaughtered annually for meat and dairy production is so large that it can only be roughly estimated to the nearest billion. In 2011, the approximate number was 70 billion land animals worldwide (Khazaal and Almiron 2016: 375). This is larger than the number of animals killed for hunting, shelters, and research combined (Brown 2011: 23). The only industry responsible for more animal deaths is the fishing industry (Safina 2018). The population of living farm animals is about four times that of humans (Khazaal and Almiron 2016: 375). Most of these animals are denied meaningful protection and treated as nothing more than machines (Perry and Brandt 2008: 118). For example, most chickens in factory farms are unable to stretch their wings, a natural behaviour for birds (Leder 2012: 73). However, despite the staggeringly high numbers involved, farming is not the area of animal harm that attracts the largest amount of human concern. Three factors contribute to this lack of concern. The first reason is speciesism; the animals involved in food farming do not score on the higher-level of the socio-zoological scale. The second reason is because of the "happy farm" myth; romantic images of animal farming generally suggest that modern farms are happy and wholesome places for animals to live at. This misleading image is frequently repeated and is often at the forefront in WDAS films set in rural narratives, as this chapter will evidence. The third reason is because farm animals are rarely individualized; this factor leads to the "collapse of compassion" effect. To summarize, speciesism, romanticism, and the "collapse of compassion" effect have resulted in the problems with animal farming being widely ignored.

[2] This chapter will focus only on the farming of land animals for food: therefore, fur farms, puppy farms, fish farms, and so forth will not be discussed in this chapter.

After the last Ice Age came the Neolithic Revolution (around 10,000 BC) in which humans changed from hunter-gatherers to farmers (Pringle 1998: 1446). During this period, humans began to settle close to each other and develop complex social bonds. These social bonds are what would subsequently become early human civilizations (Norwood and Lusk 2011: 18). As a result of farming, human societies began to produce healthier children, which allowed societies to grow much larger than they had previously, and at a much faster pace (Pringle 1998: 1446). In the past, not all regions had huge amounts of animals and land suitable for farming: therefore, early farming somewhat shaped the future wealth of many countries (Norwood and Lusk 2011: 13). Today, around 38% of the Earth's ice-free land is used for farming, with about 70–75% of this land being used to farm animals (Deckers 2016: 22).

During the past 10,000 years, most humans would have been farm workers of some kind. For example, in the fourteenth century, 76% percent of people worked in farming, but today just 26% of all workers globally work in agriculture (Van der Zee 2018). Additionally, in developed countries, this number drops even further. For example, in the UK, only 2% of people are directly employed by the farming industry (Van der Zee 2018). However, this does not mean that farming has declined; in fact, more animals than ever before are killed as part of the farming industry's routine operations. This decrease in employment is because agriculture has become industrialized; many of the jobs previously undertaken by humans are now performed by machines. Traditionally, farm animals were used to assist in farm labour, as well as to provide meat, dairy, and so forth (Leder 2012: 74). However, the rise in farm technology meant that animals were no longer needed to help with the labour; they were only needed for the products they could produce, and this shift led to the development of factory farming. The first species to be factory farmed was the chicken, then pigs, and more recently cattle (Van der Zee 2018). The increased production scale of factory farming requires that these animals live shorter lives, and also that they weigh more. For example, since 1925, the life of a farmed chicken has dropped from 112 days to 48 days, while their weight has risen from 2.5 pounds to 6.2 pounds (Van der Zee 2018). Because of this efficiency, the cost of meat and dairy has dropped considerably (Brown 2011: 23). For example, the price of chicken has decreased by 110 percent over the past fifty years (Norwood and Lusk 2011: 39–40). The efficiency of modern agriculture quickly became more profitable than the more humane, free-range, farming alternatives. However, these shifts have been detrimental for the animals involved. For example, Brown (2011) suggests that modern factory farms have no regard for the individual needs of the animals (2011: 23). This has been repeatedly demonstrated through the many exposé videos that have been produced by undercover animal rights activists (for example: *PETA* 2019f). As a result, factory farming is often compared to infamous examples of the poor treatment of humans in history, such as the prisoners in the gulags, or the way that privileged classes once colonized indigenous peoples (Plumwood 2012: 57, 72). In general, there are very few laws protecting farmed animals, and the ones that do exist are inconsistent. For instance, in America, the Humane Slaughter Act prohibits the unnecessary suffering of farmed animals, but this act excludes birds, which is problematic because more chickens are slaughtered for food per year than any other land animal (Norwood and Lusk 2011: 60–1). Thus, chickens, the most commonly-farmed species of land animal, can legally be neglected and mistreated in American farms.

As with some other forms of animal harm and objectification, humans are negatively affected by the farming industry. The majority of slaughterhouse[3] employees in America are low-paid, young, single, men (Fitzgerald et al. 2009: 160; Schlosser 2004: 149). It is claimed that large farms (also known as megafarms) are purposefully built near deprived areas, presumably to attract people who are more willing to work in poor conditions for low-wages (Deckers 2016: 16). It is noted that the rate of suicide amongst farm workers is three times the national average in America (Schlosser 2004: 146). It is also claimed that the annual staff turnover rate in the meatpacking industry is around 400 percent, with the average worker leaving or being dismissed within three months (Schlosser 2004: 160). In fact, Adams (2010) argues that the staff turnover rates amongst slaughterhouse workers are the highest of any occupation in America

[3] Factory farms and slaughterhouses are separate locations with separate purposes. Thus, they are not synonymous terms. However, almost all animals raised in factory farms will die in a slaughterhouse or similar facility (*PETA* 2019g). This is why the two locations are discussed alongside each other and often interchangeably in this chapter.

(2010: 80). Moreover, a 2018 *Guardian* article claimed that American meat plant workers are three times more likely to suffer serious injury than other US workers, with an average of two amputations per week (Wasley et al. 2018). Cumulatively, this evidence suggests that working in the modern farming industry has severely negative physical and mental effects on employees. Additionally, given the economic background of these workers, it seems likely that most employees of the modern animal farming industry work in that industry because they have few other options, and not because they have chosen to work in such a challenging environment. Singer (2009) claims that the people who kill animals in socially-acceptable ways, such as in slaughterhouses, are generally not "cruel and wicked" (Singer 2009: 97). The reality is that the jobs these people undertake are a result of normalized speciesism, rather than an intention to inflict harm for personal gratification. Given that the evidence presented here suggests that these industries have a high turnover and are purposefully built in deprived areas, Singer's claims do appear to hold merit. Despite this, cultural portrayals of those who work in slaughterhouses are often unsympathetic. To illustrate, in *The Texas Chain Saw Massacre* (1974), an antagonistic family of villainous cannibals repeatedly reference that they used to work in a slaughterhouse. Throughout the film, a connection between cannibalism, violence, and slaughterhouse work is frequently alluded to (Bernard 2011: 413–32). *Massacre* seems to suggest that the cannibal family became evil as a result of their earlier slaughterhouse employment, or perhaps that evil people are attracted to these violent industries. Thus, from either reading, the portrayal of slaughterhouse employees in *Massacre* is an unflattering and unsympathetic one. As will be discussed in Part III of this chapter, the harsh reality of farm work is far removed from WDAS's romantic portrayal of it, and this inaccuracy extends to the humans who work in these industries. WDAS commonly depicts farmers, but these tend to be nomadic or organic farmers that live harmoniously alongside a small number of pet-like farm animals. WDAS has not yet included a modern slaughterhouse worker or factory-farm worker among their large cast of characters, only organic, "free range", farmers. WDAS has, however, depicted some hunters and fishers (i.e. people who attempt to directly kill animals, sometimes for food). These characters will be discussed in the next chapter.

Despite the fact that farming has changed greatly during the past one hundred years, cultural representations of farming suggest that this practice is still aligned with its nomadic roots. Singer notes that most depictions of farms are optimistic, romantic, and far removed from the reality of most modern farming (2009: 96). Singer further claims that many people think of farms as more pleasant than "our own industrial, profit-conscious city life" (2009: 96). Misleading depictions of farms often include happy, subservient animals that are treated as willing co-workers and pets, rather than objects (Buller 2013: 159–60). Additionally, farms are rarely depicted as places where intentional killing occurs (Buller 2013: 159–60). These misleading, romantic, and unrealistic images are particularly widespread in children's media, such as storybooks (Connell 2018). For example, children's books often depict picturesque, spacious farms, occupied by a variety of happy farm animals (Newkey-Burden 2018). In reality, most modern farms only house one type of species, but in huge numbers. For example, in the UK, chickens are typically housed in artificially-lit barns with 20,000–30,000 other chickens (Lawrence 2016). Each chicken will typically have the space of a sheet of A4 paper to move and live in for most of their short life (Lawrence 2016). In addition to the culturally prevalent "happy farm" image, modern megafarms are often kept hidden from the populace by being purposefully built in areas uninhabited by humans (Plumwood 2012: 55–74; Singer 2009: 216). Moreover, the buildings themselves do not usually advertise their purpose. As a result, few people would be able to differentiate a storage barn from a broiler shed (Singer 2009: 216). Part of this attenuation is also evident in the way that meat and dairy is sold. The majority of commercially sold meat is neatly packaged and sealed (Connell 2018). This meat is sometimes dyed with a red colorant and injected with water to make it look more appealing, or perhaps more like the meat people are used to seeing in common cultural depictions (Connell 2018). This highlights that consumers are not only misled about the reality of farming, but also the reality of animal products. Perhaps because of its established romantic image, it is believed that the average person has little knowledge about the realities of modern farming (Norwood and Lusk 2011: 246, 259). This miseducation may be because of the false portrayals of animal farming fed to the public, such as those present in WDAS films.

Additionally, it is noted that the meat and dairy industries have run many high-profile advertising campaigns that promote their products as both healthy and natural. For example, the dairy industry often boasts about the apparent health and nutritional benefits of their products (Wrenn 2017: 74). However, even though these images are somewhat misleading, and in some cases incorrect, it is argued that there is much interest in keeping this romantic image alive in order to protect these profitable industries (Buller 2013: 159–60).

The romanticized "happy farm" image frequently depicted in children's media is usually set in the pre-industrialized past, as is the case with the farms in most WDAS films. However, it is unlikely that ancient farms were as ethical as the "happy farm" image suggests. As evidenced earlier, farm animals were usually required to participate in the hard labour of pre-industrial farms. This practice would likely be viewed as cruel by many today, hence why it is often omitted in depictions of nomadic farming. The reason that the "happy farm" image exists is simple: when animal harm is visible, it can drastically change how people feel about the end product. For instance, a 2013 study found that when people were shown images of animal cruelty in slaughterhouses, the most common reactions were sympathy for the animal and disgust at the situation (Tiplady et al. 2013: 869, 882). Animal rights activists have successfully used this sensitivity to further their cause (Lancaster and Boyd 2015: 186). For example, a common tactic of the modern animal rights movement is for activists to go undercover on farms, film the worst instances of cruelty that they see, and then portray it as being normal practice. Upon their release, these videos are evidently met with outrage towards the farms or equivalent. In fact, documented instances of animal harm have put many farming companies out of business (Shea 2015: 349). This type of activism has worked well to reduce consumption of certain farm products, such as veal and foie gras (Paynter 2014). For example, the production of veal, which involves keeping male calves in crates, was banned in the UK in the 1990s after many anti-veal campaigns focussed on the cruelty of this practice (Levitt 2018; Paynter 2014). Consequently, the American meat industry has recently tried to stop the production of videos and photography in their slaughterhouses and farms (Shea 2015: 349). For these reasons, some companies that use animal products, such as McDonald's, have publicly attempted to help improve farming conditions to better their own PR image (Leder 2012: 74). However, despite these points, American consumers spend more on meat than any other food category (Norwood and Lusk 2011: 204). In addition to these points, some research has noted that people who oppose the consumption of meat and dairy, such as vegans, are frequently ridiculed in the media (Cole and Morgan 2011: 134–153). Therefore, it can be concluded that most people do not want to see an end to meat consumption; they want higher standards of welfare for farm animals. However, a desire for ethical farming is somewhat illogical given that meat cannot exist without the un-consensual death of an animal (Adams 2010: 66). This problem is also partly caused by the "happy farm" image, which creates the illusion that farming does not involve death.

Even though billions of animals are slaughtered for food annually, only a select few species are used by the farming industry. In the Anglo-American context, farming mainly affects chickens, cows, pigs, and turkeys (*ASPCA* 2018).[4] This is one of the main arguments against animal farming from an animal rights viewpoint: farming is speciesist. Not all animals are capable of being domesticated, and thus farmed. Species that were able to be farmed grew quickly. Such animals are comfortable in packs, eat a mostly herbivorous diet, and are docile (Norwood and Lusk 2011: 12–3). Over time, humans have selectively bred these species to accentuate what humans have believed to be their more-useful features, such as large breasts on chickens (Schatzker 2015). However, as a result, these species have since been genetically altered by humans, and therefore would today struggle to survive without human assistance (Norwood and Lusk 2011: 8). Therefore, even if animal farming was stopped, it is unlikely that modern farm animals could ever return to their natural habitat.

---

[4] It is noted, however, that farmed species vary somewhat between cultures. For example, in India, cows are worshipped, but, in the UK, they are commonly bred for slaughter (Norwood and Lusk 2011: 20). This text is focussed on animals in the Anglo-American context as this is the location of the majority of WDAS films. Therefore, in this book, cows, pigs, and chickens are considered to be the three most commonly farmed animals (*ASPCA* 2018). Additionally, while horses often "live" on farms, they are not usually eaten in the Anglo-American world. Therefore, they will be discussed in Chap. 4 alongside working animals.

While some species, such as cats and dogs, are often individualized in WDAS films, farm animals are usually depicted in groups. However, this is problematic from an animal welfare perspective because depicting animals in larger groups can result in the "collapse of compassion" effect: thus, any harm the group undergoes might result in a less compassionate response than individual instances elicit. On the rare occasions when farm animals have been individualized in fiction, perceptions of their rights have changed. For example, *Babe* (1995) is a film that appears to have influenced some viewers' perceptions of eating meat. *Babe* is a comedy-drama about an anthropomorphised pig that dreams of being a sheep dog. During the film, Babe (the pig) escapes being slaughtered several times, often in comical circumstances. The story ends happily with Babe achieving his ambition of becoming a "sheep dog" and thus avoiding his fate as a farmed pig. In the period following the film's release, there was a dramatic rise in the number of vegetarians, especially young female vegetarians (Nobis 2009: 58). This change in attitude was dubbed the "*Babe* effect" (Nobis 2009: 58). The "*Babe* effect" likely occurred because this film depicted farm animals as intelligent, individual, and compassionate individuals, something that had seldom been done previously and is usually reserved for higher-order species (Plumwood 2012: 55–74).

Because they are purposefully built in uninhabited areas, very few people have been inside a megafarm or slaughterhouse. Most people's only experience of them is vicariously, such as through a book or film (Adams 2010: 78). While farms are often portrayed positively, *Babe* providing one example, slaughterhouses and the like are rarely presented favourably. *The Texas Chain Saw Massacre* is one such example of this point. Burt (2002) notes that the slaughterhouse image rarely appears in mainstream films. Similarly, documentary films that accurately document realistic slaughterhouses and the like are usually reviled. For example, *PETA* has produced many videos that aim to expose the harsh reality of these places (Tonsor and Widmar 2012: 59–72). Such films have often been censored, or in some cases banned outright (*PETA* 2019c). A rare exception to this is *Chicken Run* (2000), a British stop-motion animation centred around a chicken pie factory. However, in *Chicken Run*, most of the farmed chickens manage to escape from their farm unharmed before they are turned into chicken pies (Cole and Stewart 2014). The animals in *Chicken Run* spend the rest of their lives on a chicken sanctuary after successfully escaping their farm. None of the primary characters die, and the only chicken deaths mentioned are off-screen and typically involve nameless characters. Thus, while *Chicken Run* offers a slightly more realistic look at modern animal farming, its optimistic ending is unrealistic because real farmed chickens have almost no chance of escape.

To summarize, this section has demonstrated that animal farming has been a key component of human civilization for the past ten thousand years. Animal farming initially benefitted humans, but it has resulted in a massive amount of animal harm and deaths. Moreover, the species involved have had their biology permanently altered by selective breeding practices. Yet despite the many problems with modern farming, farms are typically represented in an old-fashioned romantic way in cultural representations, which has perhaps led to people being mis-educated on the realities of contemporaneous agricultural practice. This is often termed the "happy farm" myth. Only a small number of cultural representations, such as *PETA*'s exposés, have attempted to address the reality of the situation.

Part II: Data

Please see pages 125–127 for a full list of all of the individual instances of animal farming in WDAS films. In summary, WDAS has depicted dairy[5] in twenty-five films (45%),[6] eggs in twelve films (21%), meat in thirty films (54%), a farm house in fourteen films (25%), chickens in nineteen films (34%), cows in fifteen films (27%), and pigs in sixteen films (29%). In total, this means that thirty WDAS films (54%) feature a species that is usually considered a farm animal.

---

[5] This includes any product that can reasonably be considered dairy, such as milk, cheese, or ice-cream. This does not include products that often include dairy, such as pies or cakes, as dairy is not the primary ingredient of these products. Additionally, only dairy and eggs normally consumed by humans, such as chickens' eggs or cows' milk, are included. Thus, the list does not include the dinosaur eggs in *Fantasia* (1940), for example.

[6] The percentages have been rounded-up/ down to one decimal point.

Part III: Animal Farming in WDAS Films

Walt spent his early-childhood on a rural farm, which he often claimed were the best days of his life: "Those were the happiest days of my life, and maybe that's why I go in for country cartoons. Gosh, I hated to leave it" (Walt, in: Jackson 2005: 11). Roy also remembered this farm fondly and stated that it was "a very cute, sweet little farm" (Roy, in: Barrier 2007: 11). The farm itself was forty-five acres and included orchids of apples, peaches, and plums, plus fields of grain (Barrier 2007: 11). The farm also housed animals, such as hogs, chickens, horses, and cows, but it is claimed that there were only a few dozen of these animals (Barrier 2007: 11). This suggests that the farm's emphasis was on crops rather than animal products. It is clear that these fond memories affected Walt's early-animations, an influence that can still be seen throughout WDAS films today. However, Tobias (2011) argues that:

> For the Disney family, as for most Americans, farm animals were objects, devoid of subjective content. Their capacity to suffer was limited, and their duty in life was to serve. [Walt]'s barnyard humour provided the foundation for much of his early work. He relegated domesticated animals to the lowest echelon of life because he, like most Americans, considered them soulless husks, undeserving of moral consideration.

Given how favourably some animals were presented in the early Disney works, it would be unfair to agree that Walt viewed animals in the way that Tobias (2011) suggests. However, it is clear that Walt afforded much more moral consideration to certain species of animals, as this book will demonstrate. For example, higher-order species, such as dogs, have been spared negative depictions in many WDAS works, such as *Lady and the Tramp* and *Oliver & Company*. Yet Tobias (2011) is correct in claiming that some species have been largely placed in the background of Disney media, and WDAS's common depictions of farm animals as subservient characters and objects demonstrate this.

Overall, the farms, farmers, and farm animals depicted by WDAS are overly positive, optimistic, and romantic. This may be because the timeline of the Disney company corresponds with the public's own detachment from nature (Wills 2017: 114). Walt's childhood farm was undoubtedly very different from the ones that existed later in his lifetime, given that farming has become much more industrialized since 1901 (when Walt was born). It simply would not have been possible for WDAS to depict farming realistically and still appeal to mainstream film audiences. As evidenced earlier in this chapter, realistic depictions of farming are usually disliked by Anglo-American film audiences. However, while WDAS's farm animals, farms, and so forth have been unrealistic, they have not been accidental. In animation, nothing appears accidently since everything must be drawn purposefully. Thus, WDAS's depiction of farming is an intentional one, which means that its romantic nature warrants questioning.

While WDAS has ignored the negatives associated with farming (such as slaughter and factory farming), they have not neglected farms themselves. As shown in the data presented in Part II of this chapter, farms are depicted in 25% of WDAS films. WDAS's farms are usually family-run and based around family homes with free-range paddocks that house a small number of pet-like animals. Additionally, most of the farms in WDAS texts are part of a wider community and do not hide the fact that they are farming animals. As evidenced in Part I, modern factory farms are intentionally built in uninhabited areas and hide their true purpose. In contrast, WDAS's farms are proud of their existence. For example, in *The Black Cauldron* (1985), the sweet-natured protagonist Taran lives on "Caer Dallben", a little farm populated with a small number of happy free-range animals. Taran's farm is depicted as a warmly-lit, safe, and happy location for both humans and other animals. In contrast, the outside world (which Taran later travels to) is presented as dangerous and with many villainous characters. Additionally, it has also been noted that the plants on WDAS's farms are also unrealistic and somewhat romanticized. For example, Whitley (2008) notes that the crops in *Pocahontas* (1995) are unnaturally organized in straight neat rows with few insects, meaning that they resemble idealized genetically-modified crops rather than the crops that would have existed in the pre-industrial period in which *Pocahontas* is set (2008: 86). Therefore, WDAS's romanticism of farming extends beyond animals.

Despite the lack of realism in WDAS's depictions of farming, it is worth noting that critics have often praised Disney for their commitment to realism compared with their animation rivals, such as Warner Brothers and UPA (Pallant 2010b: 105–6). It is claimed that Disney's early work displayed a predominantly-abstract and non-realist form, but with verisimilitude in respect to characterization, contexts, and narratives (Wells 1998: 23). Walt wanted his characters to move realistically and be plausibly motivated (Wells 1998: 23; Pallant 2010b: 104). This form of animation continued throughout Walt's career, and by the time WDAS was founded, Walt insisted that his animators study the movements of real animals and people in order to perfect the movement and appearance of their characters (Wells 1998: 23). However, this commitment to realism has not yet extended to WDAS's portrayal of the farming industry. Additionally, this accuracy seems to only apply to the positive aspects of animal behaviour and appearance. For example, the usefulness of farm animals, such as cows providing milk, is depicted. However, the reality of modern farming, such as cows being milked via efficient machinery, is not. A slaughterhouse or similar facility has never been shown in any WDAS film. This is problematic because the farming industry kills more land animals than any other industry. Thus, WDAS is misleading their viewers by negating a large part of the modern farming industry and real farm animals' lives. Since every WDAS film features animals, it seems fair to suggest that their second most common cause of death should be acknowledged. It seems that WDAS leans towards realism when accentuating positive elements and eschews realism if it means engaging with negative elements. The same approach is evident elsewhere; WDAS often depicts overweight middle-aged male characters (such as the sultan in *Aladdin* or LeFou in *Beauty and the Beast*), but they do not regularly depict the negatives of middle-age obesity, such as heart attacks or diabetes (even though that is a commonplace reality for this demographic). Thus, WDAS seems to only ever depict the more light-hearted or romanticized elements of serious issues. This will be further evidenced in this text with analyses of pet-keeping, animal performers, and the production of fur.

Furthermore, it is clear that WDAS's commitment to realism applies to some species of animals more than others. There is no evidence of conventional farm animals being brought into Disney's animation studios for the animators to observe. However, this practice was common with other, often higher-order, animals, such as elephants (for *Dumbo*) and dogs (for *Lady and the Tramp*) (for example: Pallant 2011: 47). By not animating directly from farm animals, WDAS's representations are even further separated from the reality of modern agricultural practice. For example, it is common practice for battery chickens to be de-beaked to prevent them from pecking other animals (*BHWT* 2019). Yet the farm chickens depicted in WDAS films, such as *The Fox and the Hound* (1981) and *Home on the Range* (2004), always appear to have their beaks, and this practice is not mentioned in these narratives. Further to this, WDAS's farm animals are animated in a much simpler, less-anthropomorphised, and less-unique way than WDAS's other animal characters. For example, chickens are rarely protagonists or antagonists, nor are they usually individualized. They are usually light-hearted supporting and background characters in small groups of their species. Their appearance is usually similar to other characters of their species with few individual characteristics. In contrast, higher-order species, such as dogs, are usually designed with a distinctive appearance and individual personality, as can be seen in *Lady and the Tramp*, for example. Additionally, the farm animals in WDAS films always seem happy with their situation and never show any signs of mistreatment. Moreover, none of the animal characters that have ever died in WDAS films have been conventional farm animals, even though animal farming is the most-common killer of land animals in reality.

Singer notes that portrayals of dairy cows in cultural representations tend to be romantic even though most cows alive today have been essentially reduced to milking machines (2009: 137). In WDAS films, cows are usually depicted as being content farm animals, even when producing milk for humans or other animals. Outside of the industrial agricultural context, real cows produce milk for the nutritional benefit of their own offspring (*RSPCA* 2019b). However, there are no examples of calves drinking cows' milk in any WDAS film. In fact, no calves are depicted in any WDAS film; all of WDAS's cows are adults and never appear to be pregnant. This implies that cows' milk does not exist for calves, but for humans and other animals. For example, in *Dalmatians*, there are several anthropomorphised dairy cows that happily offer their milk to the travelling Dalmatian puppies. The cows are shown as happy to lactate for another species, and they also seem quite content in their barn. This is evinced by their grins and the statements they make, such as "I wish they [the puppies] could stay with us for always" [sic]. This suggests that the cows' only purpose in this film is to provide milk to the travelling puppies. They are not depicted before or after this scene, nor do they have calves or appear to be pregnant even though they are able to express milk. Thus, their only purpose is to provide milk when needed by other species. However, as Chap. 3 will highlight, *Dalmatians* argues that puppies are worth more than their fur, i.e. the objects their bodies can produce. This shows a clear contradiction between the errors of objectifying one species (puppies) and the social-acceptance of objectifying another (cows). This is because the production of milk is socially-acceptable, whereas the production of fur is not.

A similar argument can be made for the way in which WDAS has depicted chickens. Connell (2018) argues that the scrawny mutilated chicken could serve as a mascot for the reality of factory farming. This is because around 80% of all meat produced is chicken flesh, meaning that more chickens are killed in the production of food than any other land animal (Deckers 2016: 54). Somewhat accurately, chickens are also WDAS's most commonly-depicted farm animal. However, there are zero instances of chicken slaughter in any WDAS films; thus, WDAS is again ignoring the uncomfortable reality of modern animal farming. This is problematic because WDAS's output negates the reason why most chickens exist: the species' existence is almost solely defined by humans using their bodies (consuming their flesh or the eggs they produce). Evidence suggests that many people believe that chickens are happy with their lives. For example, an American study found that 71% of people believe that free-range hens are happy and content (Norwood and Lusk 2011: 247). This suggests that many people are unaware of how far removed farm animals are from their natural living conditions. Most chickens spend their lives in wire cages in windowless "barns" (Norwood and Lusk 2011: 247). These aspects of chickens' lives are rarely represented in culture, and certainly never in WDAS films even though chickens are such common characters. 34% of WDAS films feature chickens, but only in free-range situations far removed from the lives that most chickens experience. For example, *The Fox and the Hound* (1981) includes a single hen nesting with her three chicks in Widow Tweed's barn. This hen is seen smiling and looks comfortable in her roomy nest. In this respect, WDAS has helped to sustain a notion that hens are content with their role in the agricultural setting. Even Amos Slade, the film's fox-hating antagonist, has a large outdoor pen and hen house for his small brood of chickens. Thus, in WDAS films, even the villains treat farm animals kindly. The example above also demonstrates how farm animals are less-anthropomorphised than the other species in the same text. In *The Fox and the Hound*, the fox (Tod) and Copper (the dog) can speak and express many human-like facial emotions. In contrast, the nameless chicken and her nameless chicks do not speak.

Additionally, WDAS's jolly farmers are far removed from contemporary farm workers. From Johnny Appleseed in *Melody Time* to Pearl Gesner in *Home on the Range*, WDAS's farmers are optimistic and wholesome characters with no interest in harming animals. It is usually the case that WDAS's farmers live in a farm house with their animals performing pet-like roles. For example, in *The Fox and the Hound* (1981), Widow Tweed is a jolly elderly woman who lives in a bungalow with a barn outside. In her barn, she has a small number of individualized farm animals whom she personally farms in a compassionate way. For example, she is seen gently milking and talking to her pet cow Abigail. Later, she is shown hugging Abigail after Tod scares her. This conflation of home and farm connotes that the cow-human relationship is semi-familial. Even if there is an inbuilt hierarchy, the cow and human co-exist in a productive way: it is not that the cow is purely of instrumental value to the human. The situation also contrasts with the now typical geography of contemporary agriculture – which happens far from the consumer's everyday context. Thus, WDAS's depiction of farmers is in stark contrast to the reality of most farm workers today. Part I presented evidence that most modern farm workers do work that is both mentally and physically challenging; additionally, they have little chance for bonding with individual animals because of the sheer numbers and short lives of the animals involved.

Meat and dairy are often evident in WDAS films, but the intense farming required to generate those foods is rarely depicted. Cows are occasionally milked in WDAS films, but this has never been depicted as cruel or unnatural. Whenever WDAS has shown cows producing milk, the cows are happy to do so. Similarly, only once have chickens been shown laying eggs (*Home on the Range*). As highlighted in Part II of this chapter, 54% of the WDAS films in this study feature some kind of meat, and 54% feature a common farm animal. However, these instances do not always coincide. Some films that feature meat or dairy, such as *Atlantis* (2001), do not feature any farm animals. Similarly, some films that include common farm animals, such as *Winnie the Pooh* (2011), feature no farm products at all. This again demonstrates the disconnection between farm animals and animals as food. It implies that the two are separate, even though meat and dairy cannot exist without farm animals. Despite this separation, WDAS's portrayal of meat-eaters is unflattering and not romanticized at all.

Adams claims that patriarchal structures promote the idea that meat is masculine (2010: 48, 56). For example, physically-strong, heavily-muscular men, such as wrestlers and weight-lifters, are commonly portrayed as heavy meat eaters (Adams 2010: 56–7). Moreover, men who abstain from meat eating are often perceived as un-masculine (Adams 2010: 57). This idea is echoed in WDAS films. For example, the overtly-masculine Gaston in *Beauty and the Beast* (1991) proudly boasts about his high meat and raw egg intake to other, less-muscly, men. Gaston has a large physique, brags about his hunting achievements, and even has his own eponymous song that celebrates his many manly features. Gaston's henchman LeFou compliments him by telling him that: "No beast alive stands a chance against you, and no girl for that matter". Another example of this characterization is found in 1963s *The Sword and the Stone* (1963), in which the spoilt and brutish Sir Kay is seen eating enormous amounts of meat after his knighthood training. This example also suggests that eating large amounts of meat produces more muscle. This connotation is about mastery and control over the self (training), but also an exertion of power over animal flesh. Animal flesh is there to become part of his flesh, to improve him – he possesses it. As he eats large amounts of meat, Kay boasts about how little he cares about Arthur, whom he refers to as "the wart". This slur, alongside the large amounts of greasy meat around him, portrays Kay as an insensitive character. It again suggests, as

Adams (2010) highlights, that meat-eaters are toxically masculine.[7] These men are insensitive to the processes involved in creating meat (death), and although the films seem critical of their insensitivity, the films are also complicit in negating those processes. In cultural representations, harming animals is often an indicator of a villainous character, so it makes sense that meat eating also indicates this because the production of meat always involves animal death (Arluke 2006: 3).

In contrast to this, WDAS's male characters that do not eat meat are portrayed as somewhat feminine. For instance, Johnny Appleseed in *Melody Time* (1948) is a skinny gentle unmarried man, who seems to only eat and farm apples and is never depicted eating any animal products or farming animals for food. There are animals in his narrative, but Johnny does not use or harm them. To refer back to quote at the beginning of the chapter, it is worth noting that in *Fun and Fancy Free*, the starving farmers Mickey, Goofy, and Donald do not eat meat when they arrive at the giant's castle, even though they are starving, and it is freely available to them. Instead, the three pro-social farmers feast on peas and jelly. In contrast, the insensitive oafish giant eats chicken ungraciously, which immediately establishes him as a villainous character. By depicting toxically-masculine men as meat consumers, and gentlemen as herbivores, WDAS implies that the consumption of meat is associated with villainy and toxic-masculinity. However, connecting meat-eating with antagonistic characters is inaccurate given that most humans today, male and female, eat meat (*The Vegan Society* 2019). Therefore, it is clear that WDAS's inaccurate portrayal of farming also extends to the products created on farms, such as meat.

It is also notable that most of WDAS's meat-eating animals are also villainous. For example, in *The Lion King*, Scar feeds a large chunk of zebra meat to his villainous hyena minions. The mixed-gendered group of hyenas eat this meat aggressively, animalistically, and ungraciously, even though they are heavily-anthropomorphised in many other ways. They bend over the carcass, chomp quickly, and then talk with their mouths full. This action adds to the unforgiving and insensitive character

[7] This book understands that "toxic-masculinity" is when men suppress emotions, mask distress, maintain an appearance of hardness, and use violence as an indicator of power (Salam 2019).

that the hyenas display elsewhere in the film, such as when they attempt to kill Simba. In fact, at the end of the film, the hyenas turn on Scar and appear to eat him (off-screen) after he falls from a cliff. Unlike the hyenas, the pro-social lions in the film are never seen eating meat, despite the fact that lions are carnivorous animals in reality (although Simba is shown to reluctantly eat some non-anthropomorphised insects as he adapts to life in the jungle). Therefore, it seems that meat symbolizes villainy in animal characters as well as human characters.

It is clear from both the data in Part II and the points raised in this section that WDAS has often depicted animal farming, but in a romantic way that does not reflect the harsh reality of modern agricultural practices. WDAS's farms are happy, wholesome places, inhabited by content, servile animals and considerate human farmers. This depiction perhaps originated from Walt's own idealistic farm experience, which was evidently a pre-industrialised haven seen through the naive eyes of a child and subsequently a nostalgic gaze. On WDAS's farms, there is never any mistreatment or slaughter, which is the reality for almost-all farm animals today. Thus, despite their modern prevalence, modern megafarms and slaughterhouses are simply not part of WDAS's rendition of farming. Furthermore, WDAS's depictions of meat and dairy consumers are typically negative in tone. WDAS seems to associate meat-consumption with two types of character: toxically-masculine men and villains. However, this does not reflect the reality of modern western Anglo-American consumers, most of whom eat meat. Furthermore, consuming meat is not a socially-unacceptable act in reality, despite being portrayed negatively in WDAS films. These observations are further evident with a close examination of 2004s *Home on the Range*, a Neo-Disney[8] WDAS film set on a pre-industrial dairy farm.

[8] The Neo-Disney period (2000–2008) was an experimental Disney period that included eleven films (*Fantasia 2000 – Bolt*). During the Neo-Disney period, WDAS moved away from the hand-drawn animation they had become famous for and started making animation using CGI-technology (Pallant 2010b: 104). There were several other changes too, many of which have since been abandoned. For example, the Neo-Disney films did not use music as most popular WDAS films do, i.e. with characters singing. Instead, they used montage and background music (Pallant 2010b: 110).

Part IV: Animal Farming and *Home on the Range*

As the beginning of Part I demonstrated, the reality of animal farming industry is quite gruesome. However, as the end of Part I demonstrated, and Part III of this chapter indicated, WDAS only depicts romantic images of animal farming. Therefore, it seems that despite the negative aspects of modern agriculture, this chapter will have the happy ending that WDAS films are famous for. The story of *Home on the Range* is a WDAS original, rather than being based on external texts (Singer 2004). *Range* is about a trio of female dairy cows that attempt to capture a cattle rustler who wants to buy their dairy farm. All of the villains are human, and most of the heroes are animals, which could serve as a metaphor for the dairy industry. As shown in Part I, the dairy industry is often labelled as cruel because of its inattention to animal welfare. Thus, in reality, humans *are* the "villains" of the dairy industry. However, this metaphor is where the reality of dairy farming ends with *Range*.

The film opens with a hot branding iron (the type that brands cattle) stamping the iconic Disney logo onto parchment. This opening seems to minimize what is a common way of harming farm animals. During this moment, there are no cattle on screen, and the music playing is country-western style. Because there are no cattle and the music is upbeat, cattle-branding is not depicted as a practice that is painful or which metaphorically objectifies cattle. Thus, branding irons are disconnected from their usual use and instead depicted as harmless objects that stamp parchment, not animals.

The dairy farm that *Range* centres around is sweetly named "Little Patch of Heaven". This farm offers a saccharine portrayal of farm life. When the film opens, a jolly opening song "*Little Patch of Heaven*" plays over an opening montage to introduce the location, and to exemplify the happy attitude the farm encapsulates:

> Everything's green
> Know what I mean
> Darlin' it's quite the sweetest sight that you ever done seen

Ain't nothin' much out there.
Just life at its best
On that little patch of heaven
Way out west [sic]

These lyrics establish that the farm is a happy, peaceful, and natural location that is safe for animals, and this is indeed confirmed by the narrative. The story of *Range* begins with Maggie, an ex-show cow, being sold to "Little Patch of Heaven", a transaction that she is happy with. Maggie's previous owner (Mr. Dixon) had to sell Maggie after his cattle herd was stolen by Slim, the film's villain. Upon seeing "Little Patch of Heaven", Maggie grins and states that: "I hope it's not one of them fat-free places". By referencing "fat-free", Maggie shows an understanding of how dairy products are sold outside of animal farms today. This is humorous because real dairy cows almost certainly have little understanding of the products made from their milk. This is the first of many jokes made about the modern farming industry, even though the film is set in the past. For example, Maggie proclaims: "Yeah, they're real. Quit staring!" in reference to her prize-winning udders. These jokes allude to the reality of modern animal objectification, but in a way that children are unlikely to understand. It was because of these crude jokes that *Range* was given a PG rating, which is unusual for a WDAS film (*IMDB* 2018c). These jokes seem to exist in lieu of realistic depictions of modern agriculture. Further to this, the film's subtle jokes also (perhaps more significantly) demonstrate that the film is not entirely blind to contemporary agricultural practices, and it expects the audience to share in that awareness (since the jokes rely on that awareness).

Upon her arrival at the farm, Maggie describes the farm as "heaven", "green", and "roomy". This is further confirmed by the visuals of the film. The farm is first shown through a wide camera angle, making it look large and spacious. Also, given that there are only a small number of animals living there, every animal has a generous amount of space to themselves. Each farm animal on "Little Patch of Heaven" has an individual name and personality. For example, there is an elderly grumpy goat named Jeb that collects tin cans. Because the animal characters are individualized, the "collapse of compassion" effect does not occur. Thus, when the trio of dairy cows later face danger and misfortune, the film encourages sympathy through their individual pain.

The farm is decorated with various fruit trees and sweetcorn plants, which is an uncontroversial type of farming to depict (compared with battery chicken farming, for instance). During the farm's introductory song, the cows help Pearl (the farmer) to collect fruit from the trees. Pearl does all the farming with just the help of her subservient farm animals. She has no machines or human workers to aid her, nor does she seem to need them. For example, Mrs. Calloway, one of the main cow characters, uses her flowery hat to help collect eggs from the hens. This scene implies that "Little Patch of Heaven" has a leisurely pace of life, which contrasts hugely with the inhumane efficiency of modern agriculture. Furthermore, most of the animals are depicted eating within the first five minutes of the film, implying that they are well-fed, and thus well-cared for.

Pearl, the human farm owner, is a loving, kind, elderly lady who clearly loves her farm animals and refers to them as her "family". After the opening song, it transpires that "Little Patch of Heaven" is in serious debt due to a bad harvest. This again suggests that the farm's emphasis is on selling crops rather than animal products. However, Pearl refuses to sell her livestock to save her farm on the basis that her animals are her family. She even aggressively threatens the sheriff with a hoe after he suggests it. Thus, the farm animals are clearly treated like pets rather than products by the farmer. Most of the harm the farm animals later face is a result of their own choices and jokes rather than harms inflicted by the human characters. In reality, farmed animals are directly and indirectly harmed by humans, through no fault of their own.

In addition to the subtle jokes about modern farming throughout the film, the way that the cattle are controlled by the film's villain Alameda Slim is also comedic rather than violent. Alameda Slim, the film's human cattle-rustling antagonist, uses yodelling to hypnotize the cattle into following his commands. Slim uses no cattle prods, branding irons, and so forth. Again, the lack of violence or inhumane farming tools is not reflective of how many cattle are treated by humans in reality. Slim was voiced by Randy Quaid, a famous American comedy actor (Collin 2017). This seems to further confirm that WDAS envisioned the character as humorous, rather than terrifying. Despite this humour, Slim and his gang are described by Maggie (the cow) as "The meanest bunch of cattle rustlers in the west" before they even appear on screen. The trio of farm cows try to find Slim in order to claim the $750 reward for his capture and pay off their farm's debt. People who directly harm animals are often vilified both in WDAS films and other cultural representations. However, despite his role as a cattle rustler, Slim never harms any animals, only humans. For example, he often hits his hapless (human) nephews when they do not do as he asks, or when they misunderstand his commands. It is clear that Slim does not value farm animals as dearly as Pearl does, but it could not be said that he harms, neglects, or mistreats the cattle in any way. If Slim did harm the cattle, it would likely detract from his engaging comedic character.

The human villains are easily outwitted by the farm animals, suggesting that the farm animals are equally, if not more, intelligent than humans. The film also suggests that farm animals feel pain, prejudice, love, and friendship. Thus, these farm animals are depicted as sentient and capable of feeling pain. The fact that *Range* depicts violence towards humans as justifiable, and violence towards farm animals as unethical, seems to indirectly suggest that farm animals do not deserve to be harmed. Thus, *Range* opposes factory farming, albeit indirectly. What little violence is included in the film is frequently perpetrated by animals rather than humans. For example, Patrick (the horse) and the cows defeat several human cowboys with a whip during the climax of the film. This scene ends with several of the cowboys being tied up. This sequence inverts the normal function of whips, which are typically used to control horses and livestock. However, this scene is problematic because it presents the dichotomy between humans and farm animals as a fair fight, with the animals having an equal chance of winning. In reality, farm animals have little chance to "fight back" against their mistreatment because they are usually caged and do not have access to weapons.

However, *Range* is not entirely without violence towards animals. After the film's opening shot, a wild rabbit (aptly named "Lucky Jack") is chased by a snarling grey wolf. Lucky Jack falls into a cactus and is then viciously pecked by a flock of owls. Subsequently, he is caught by a rattle snake and carried off-camera. This narrative continues throughout the film, often as a way of opening scenes. For example, Lucky Jack appears later in the film with a peg-leg, suggesting that the rattle snake was partially successful in its attempt to eat him. This violence occurs in the wilder locations, beyond the farm's boundaries, contrasting with the calm, non-violent, lives that the farm animals on the dairy farm enjoy. If Lucky Jack lived on "Little Patch of Heaven", he would be shielded from physical harm. Additionally, the farm animals in *Range* only experience harm when they are not on their farm, suggesting that farms are safer for animals than their natural environments. In fact, Jeb (the farm's goat) declares that the cows are "stew meat" as they leave the farm, further suggesting that farms are less-dangerous for cows than the outside world. This situation is the opposite of reality for most farm animals. Moreover, this depiction of farms as sanctuaries from violence is problematic given that contemporary farms are locations in which animals routinely undergo harm during meat and dairy production.

Range romanticizes the way animals were farmed before the industrial revolution, and indeed appears to be set in that pre-industrial era. The inclusion of wagons and steam trains suggest that it is set at the beginning of the Industrial Revolution. The film could not have realistically been set in the contemporary era given that this type of farm rarely exists in Anglo-American cultures today (Khazaal and Almiron 2016: 374–91). In fact, most of WDAS's farms – such as those depicted in *The Fox and the Hound* (1981), *The Black Cauldron* (1985), and *Beauty and the Beast* (1991) – appear to be set in the past. By setting their farms mostly in the past, WDAS is ignoring the real issues that affect the majority of living farm animals today. However, WDAS films can affect how people view and treat animals and animal products in reality. This will be later demonstrated with *Bambi* and *Dalmatians*, for example. Therefore, WDAS should care about their depictions of animal farming because they have the potential to improve it.

To summarize, *Range* is problematic because of its happy protagonists, idealized locations, crass jokes, and non-violent villains. The film's narrative centres around three dairy cows keeping their farm open to benefit themselves and their kind, animal-loving, owner Pearl. In *Range*, farm animals are treated like pets rather than products. Most of the objectification they face is metaphorical; it is a result of their own jokes rather than the human characters. Additionally, the direct harm they face is a result of their own choices; if the animals stayed on their dairy farm, they would not have experienced any physical harm. *Range* demonstrates how WDAS frequently minimizes, attenuates, and negates animal abuse, yet still portrays animal farming. *Range* does indirectly challenge farming, yet in a way that is too subtle to be impactful. Thus, WDAS benefits from using animals, yet animals themselves do not. Like other Neo-Disney films, *Home on the Range* (2004) broke many of WDAS's artistic and narrative traditions, but it also reinforced many too, one of which being an idealistic view of farm life. However, perhaps because of its deviation from WDAS's norms, it was not as financially successful as most other WDAS films, and it is actually considered one of their worst by both critics and viewers (*Rotten Tomatoes* 2019).

Conclusion

Farm animals have provided humans with much more than food: they have helped shape human civilization (Norwood and Lusk 2011: 32). However, while animal farming may have initially benefitted humans, it is today problematic for both humans and other animals. There are billions of farm animals in existence, almost-all of which will live uncomfortable lives and be unceremoniously killed. However, most people are unaware of, or perhaps in denial about, how these billions of animals live and die (Freeman 2009: 79). Most people do not experience farms or slaughterhouses first-hand, and so they rely upon these cultural representations as a source of knowledge.

At the time of writing, there are several new farm laws and practices on the horizon that may further impinge on the welfare of farm animals. For example, a new program in North America aims to increase slaughter speeds and recruit fewer safety inspectors (David 2018). However, at the same time, the numbers of people adopting vegan diets (and thus avoiding farm products altogether) are rising swiftly (Hancox 2018). These changes will likely put media companies such as WDAS in a difficult position. As demonstrated here, WDAS tends to depict what is socially-acceptable. This is why they have avoided depicting the production of veal or foie gras, i.e. forms of animal farming that have become socially-unacceptable, for example. Thus, if animal farming does become socially-unacceptable, then WDAS is likely to follow this trend, which would be a significant deviation from their norm. Indeed, there are some small signs that Disney is aware of the shifting attitudes towards farming. In *Moana* (2016), one of WDAS's most-recent films, the protagonist (Moana) has a pet pig sidekick named Pua and a pet chicken named Hei Hei. As with WDAS's other farm animals, Pua and Hei Hei are not as anthropomorphised as WDAS's other animal characters. For example, they are both mute and do not wear clothing. However, this is one of the first times WDAS has characterized farm animals in a non-farm role. Additionally, the film subtly acknowledges the fate of most chickens and pigs today. Moana is clearly embarrassed after eating pork and commenting on its good taste in front of Pua the pig. This highlights that pork is sourced from pigs, which had seldom been acknowledged by WDAS previously. This suggests that WDAS is responding to changes in attitudes towards farming and farm animals. *Moana* does not challenge the common mistreatment that farm animals experience, but its depiction of them as more than subservient machines is an improvement on many of WDAS's previous depictions of farm animals. This suggests that WDAS is slowly re-considering their depictions of animal farming, which could significantly improve some of the lives of the seventy billion animals that are killed on farms every year.

2

Hunting and Fishing in WDAS Films

On July 1st, 2015, Walter Palmer paid around $50,000 to hunt and kill Cecil, a male lion, in Zimbabwe (Goldman 2016; Kassam and Glenza 2015). Palmer had acted legally, yet his actions sparked a worldwide moral outrage. To illustrate, Cecil's death was mentioned over 94,000 times in print media in the three months afterwards (Bekoff 2018). This was believed to be the largest ever public response to wildlife conservation (Goldman 2016). Prior to Cecil's death, Zimbabwe had been a popular location for trophy hunters like Palmer; however, after Cecil's death, there was a sharp reduction in this type of tourism, which has since been dubbed the "Cecil effect". In 2016, it was estimated that around six-hundred lions died from trophy hunting annually; today, this number is believed to be even lower because of the "Cecil effect" (Hance 2016). Yet, in the grand scheme of annual animal deaths, six-hundred seems relatively insignificant. For example, as the previous chapter highlighted, it is estimated that seventy billion land animals are killed for the production of food every year. There are three key reasons why the death of Cecil caused so much outrage. First, Cecil was a lion, which is a higher-order species. Second, hunting, especially trophy hunting by westerners, is a type of direct animal harm that has become socially-unacceptable. Third,

R. R. Stanton, *The Disneyfication of Animals*, The Palgrave Macmillan Animal Ethics Series, https://doi.org/10.1007/978-3-030-49316-5_2

since this incident involved just one animal, it did not elicit the "collapse of compassion" response. Furthermore, Cecil had a name and well-documented backstory, which individualized him (*Oxford University* 2017). This further prohibited the "collapse of compassion" from occurring.

This chapter will discuss and analyse WDAS's depictions of hunting and fishing.[1] Hunting and fishing are analogous practices; they both involve tracking and usually directly killing an animal. However, they differ according to the species involved, context, and social acceptance. Hunting generally affects small groups of wild animals, such as birds and mammals. Fishing affects large numbers of marine life, but mostly fish, which score low on the socio-zoological scale. Part I of this chapter will explore the history and current debates surrounding these two practices. Then, Part II will look at the number of times these practices have been depicted in WDAS films. Next, Part III will explore how WDAS has portrayed hunting and fishing. Finally, Part IV will concentrate on how hunting and fishing are portrayed in 2003's *Brother Bear*. This chapter will conclude by arguing that analyses of hunting and fishing offer a direct example of common speciesist attitudes through the disparate ways that the public reacts to these two similar practices. Additionally, WDAS has helped to sustain these speciesist attitudes with their own texts. Since many types of hunting are no longer socially-acceptable, hunting is rarely romanticized. However, when it is committed by indigenous people, it is often responded to as if it is acceptable. This disparity is true both in WDAS films and the wider media, as will be highlighted in Parts I and IV of this chapter. In contrast, fishing is rarely romanticized, except occasionally as a relaxing past time for higher-order species. This is because fish score so low on the socio-zoological scale that the harms they experience do not need to be romanticized. In fact, WDAS's representations of fishing imply that fish are objects rather than sentient animals.

[1] Hunting involves directly capturing and often killing an animal (Duffy 2010: 83). The products of hunting, such as meat and fur, are indirect types of animal harm and will be further discussed in other chapters. Fishing is usually a direct form of animal harm, but it can also be indirect when machinery is used. This chapter will only discuss direct fishing as WDAS has never depicted fish farming.

Part I: The History of Hunting and Fishing[2]

In the past, hunting was a necessity for most humans; humans that did not hunt would find survival much harder; this is why humans developed a hunting instinct (Nelson et al. 2005: 396). Unlike many other forms of animal harm, hunting is not a practice unique to humans. Many other animals, such as felines, canines, and other primates also hunt (Norwood and Lusk 2011: 9). What set humans apart from other animal hunters were their tools, and that they learned to cook meat. It is believed that hunting had several positive effects on human evolution. For example, it is thought that humans became bipedal as a result of carrying hunting tools and weapons (Cartmill 1996: 9). However, since humans invented weapons and tools, they did not have the same incentive to develop the superior hunting instincts other species, such as felines, exhibit (Cartmill 1996: 12). There are various reasons why people hunt, such as food, pest-control, population control, environmental protection, and amusement (Scruton 2002: 543). These reasons change according to the time period, location, and local environment. For example, before the advent of farming, hunting was a necessity for survival, but today this is no longer the case in some parts of the world. The social acceptance of hunting seems to depend upon the reason for hunting, the species hunted, and the people hunting. To illustrate, it is unlikely that Walter Palmer would have attracted such a strong backlash after killing Cecil the lion if he had been subsistence hunting rather than trophy hunting.

Serpell (1999) argues that, contrary to popular belief, many ancient civilizations treated animals ethically. For example, in the Ancient Agrarian civilizations, such as Ancient Greece and Egypt, the unnecessarily killing of an animal was commensurate to manslaughter (1999: 44). Serpell further argues that in traditional "hunter-gatherer" settings, the respectful hunter (i.e. one that did not make the animal suffer) was seen

[2] This chapter will only consider past research directly relevant to WDAS films. It will not provide comprehensive analyses of hunting and fishing. A detailed overview of the history of human hunting is given in Matt Cartmill's 1996 text *A View to a Death in the Morning: Hunting and Nature through History*. A thorough analysis of modern poaching is given in Rosaleen Duffy's 2010 text *Nature Crime: How We're Getting Conservation Wrong*. Additionally, the history of human fishing can be found in: Brian Fagan's 2018 book *Fishing: How the Sea Fed Civilization*.

as a better hunter (1999: 41–2). However, when humans began to farm (around 10,000 years ago), they no longer needed to hunt as much. This change from hunter-gatherers to farmers is believed to have made humans less-ethical hunters (Nelson et al. 2005: 396). As highlighted above, ancient humans were believed to have held a close affinity and respect for the animals they tracked and ate. However, because wild nature can negatively affect the production of farms, it is believed that humans became less-sympathetic towards wildlife as they became better farmers. For example, animals that ate food crops were, and still are, culled (Nelson et al. 2005: 396). Resultantly, hunting has become increasingly controversial since farming became a more sustainable way of producing food. Therefore, the social-acceptance of hunting has been declining ever since humans began farming. By the 1990s, less than 10% of Americans over the age of sixteen hunted (Mechling 2004: 69–70). The majority of hunting takes place in rural areas away from cities, with deer being the most commonly hunted animals in America (Zencey 1987: 59). Thus, unlike other forms of animal harm, hunting has not changed much along with the rise in technology, except perhaps for the weapons used.

Hunting has been a widely-discussed issue within animal rights discourse. A study in 1996 found that 25% of Americans opposed hunting, which is more significant than the opposition to some other forms of animal harm, as the other chapters of this book will demonstrate (Hastings 1996: 53–9). However, as with other areas of animal harm, there is an inconsistent application of the underlying ethical principle to this opposition. For example, while many people oppose the wealthy Anglo-Americans trophy hunters that hunt endangered animals in Africa (such as Walter Palmer), people generally find it challenging to criticize the subsistence hunting practiced by indigenous people (for example: Randhawa 2017). This is because, as with other areas of animal harm, hunting is viewed in a speciesist way by the public; furthermore, views on this practice often change depending on the demographics of the humans involved. To illustrate, animal rights campaigners have occasionally been accused of racism when criticizing native or indigenous practices, particularly hunting and fishing (Beinart 1995: 11).[3] In recent years, it has been argued that indigenous people have inherent rights over their traditional territories, and thus should be exempted from legal restrictions implemented by Anglo-American cultures (Simon 2009: 405). This exception includes their right to hunt, fish, and trap animals (Simon 2009: 418). This is because it is argued that wildlife hunting is part of the cultural identity and subsistence of many indigenous people (Luz et al. 2015: 382). For example, some indigenous cultures teach hunting and fishing as part of their schooling (Luz et al. 2015: 382). However, in contrast to this, some animal rights campaigns have been accused of ignorance for promoting the idea that indigenous people live harmoniously with nature (Beinart 1995: 11). Many seem to hold the idea that all indigenous hunting is subsistence hunting, which is not always the case. For example, even though native Canadians hunt nomadically, they often sell their pelts to auction houses (Beinart 1995: 11). This is relevant because it demonstrates why different demographics are judged by different standards. If hunting is immoral per se, then that immorality should surely apply to all acts of hunting, regardless of the species hunted or the hunter's identity. This inconsistent application of the underlying ethical principle can also be seen in WDAS films, as Part III will demonstrate.

Another inconsistent application of the underlying ethical principle applies to the species hunted. For example, from 2015 to 2018, over four hundred domestic cats were dismembered and decapitated in South London (Dodd 2018). This was initially believed to be the work of a human trapping and killing the cats. The police investigation later concluded that the cats were killed by foxes; however, many of the cats' owners have not accepted this explanation (Yeginsu 2018). These deaths caused a moral panic in the neighbourhoods affected and wider country;

---

[3] In the mid-1980s, this issue turned violent in Canada when the Canadian aboriginals carried out organized attacks on environmental and animal rights groups. This was after animal rights activists successfully campaigned against the clubbing of baby seals, which led to a ban on seal pelts by the European Economic Community. The indigenous people affected were later awarded an exemption, but the export market still collapsed by 97%. This led to what was described as a "cultural breakdown" in the Inuit community: rates of domestic violence, suicide, drug abuse, welfare payments, and alcoholism rose sharply. *Greenpeace* later clarified that they were not in conflict with any indigenous groups and later argued that indigenous people should be excepted from some modern laws (Beinart 1995: 11).

this led to many of the cat-owners impacted to set up their own vigilante group. This passionate response clearly demonstrates that hunting domestic cats is socially-unacceptable in the UK. However, the hunting of other species in the UK receives little criticism, press attention, and police time, which again highlights the speciesism of the issue. For example, even though it is illegal to hunt foxes with dogs in the UK, fox hunting with dogs is evidenced to still take place regularly, with the police being aware, yet not enforcing the laws (Agerholm 2018).

Furthermore, one of the reasons why poaching[4] garners so much attention is because of the species involved, which are often physically-large, highly-ranked species, such as elephants, lions, and rhinos. These species are frequently depicted as being entitled to their natural environment and behaviours, unlike other commonly hunted and farmed animals, such as chickens and fish. For example, common images of elephants come mostly from wildlife programmes, animation, films, and books, in which they are depicted as majestic creatures, undeserving of the harm they sometimes receive (Duffy 2010: 129). This is also how they are depicted in WDAS films, such as *The Jungle Book*, *The Lion King*, and *Tarzan*. However, most Anglo-American people have not seen elephants in their natural habitats exhibiting their natural, often-destructive, behaviours, which means that cultural representations of elephants are perhaps romanticized, and thus misleading (Duffy 2010: 153).

While the hunting of animals by humans is seen by many as unacceptable, animal-on-animal hunting is largely seen as natural and thus acceptable. For example, in the UK, household cats are responsible for the deaths of approximately 175 million animals annually, mostly birds and rodents (Scruton 2002: 561). However, these 175 million animal deaths are rarely commented upon; thus, the public clearly accept it. As highlighted above, the hunting of domestic cats was met with outrage, but the continual hunting of wildlife by domestic cats attracts little attention. In fact, carnivorous animals (i.e. animals that hunt) are usually higher-order species that are protected from being hunted by humans. For example,

[4] Poaching is defined as the *illegal* hunting of any animal (Duffy 2010: 83). It can also include fishing, collecting birds' eggs, and even buying banned animal products such as ivory and tiger bones (Duffy 2010: 86). This means that poaching is a subset of both hunting and fishing.

when Walter Palmer hunted Cecil, there was much public outrage over Cecil's death. However, given that Cecil was a lion, he likely hunted many animals himself, which was not dwelt upon in the commentary surrounding the incident. It seems that even though humans have a natural instinct for hunting, it is today not socially-acceptable for them to act upon it, which contrasts from how people treat other animals that instinctively hunt. This inconsistency may be because of the widespread misconception that humans are not animals (McPhedran 2009). This may be why hunting, an act commonly practiced by non-human animals, is seen as animalistic, and thus socially-unacceptable, for humans.

While hunting for food and clothing was a common ancient practice, trophy hunting (the slaughtering of large wild animals) has always been less common, probably because it is much more dangerous for the hunters and involves animals that are sometimes inedible. In Africa, trophy hunting is rooted in both colonialism and patriarchy given that it is practiced predominantly by wealthy white males (Weisberger 2017). However, it is also worth noting that trophy hunting, like purchasing fur and ivory, is too expensive for most people to practice. For example, Walter Palmer's trip to Zimbabwe in which he killed Cecil cost around $50,000 (Weaver and Gajanan 2015). Thus, the majority (with an average income or less) cannot afford to indulge in these practices. Thus, since these practices are only engaged with by a minority, they are not normative by default. In contrast, consuming meat, practising fishing, and wearing leather are much more affordable, and these practices are all socially-acceptable. This suggests that trophy hunting is more vilified than local wildlife hunting because of the wealth disparity it exemplifies. This point will be further expanded upon in Chap. 3 with fur, leather, and other products made from animals' bodies.

Given the importance of hunting throughout human evolution and history, it has often been depicted and documented in art, literature, mythologies, and so forth (Van der Zee 2018). The visual media has attempted to televise real hunting, but with little success (Zencey 1987: 60). Because of this, it is noted that there are few famous hunters, which is in contrast to most other sports (Zencey 1987: 62). In fact, the most famous, or rather infamous, hunters are probably ones from cultural representations, such as the faceless men in *Bambi*, Disney's Davy Crockett, or the often-shamed real ones on social media. Hunting as a practice is seldom seen in full (both in fiction and reality) because it takes place over long periods of time. This means that most people only see hunters before and after they hunt, which creates a set, and perhaps misleading, image of this practice (Zencey 1987: 60). Since many people oppose hunting, it is perhaps unsurprising that cultural representations of hunters are typically unflattering. This is consistent with other types of characters that harm or objectify animals in ways that are socially-unacceptable, such as slaughterhouse workers and fur-wearers. Hunters are often stereotyped as being insensitive, misogynistic, violent, insecure, and heavy-drinkers (Zencey 1987: 63). One famous example of this is in Golding's *Lord of the Flies* (1954). In this text, a group of school boys hunt and kill a boar after becoming standard on a desert island. After the incident, the boys become noticeably more violent and aggressive towards each other (Golding 1954). Therefore, *Lord of the Flies* strongly suggests a direct link between hunting animals and hunting humans. Certainly, in WDAS films, direct animal harm, such as hunting, is often depicted as unacceptable, abnormal, and is usually associated with villainous characters. Despite this, in reality, hunting is committed by various demographics of people for different reasons. This is similar to the points raised in the previous chapter in that fictional meat-eaters are often depicted unfavourably in WDAS films, yet in reality, meat is eaten by most humans.

To summarize the first section of Part I, it is clear that hunting is viewed negatively, but this negativity depends on the species, time period, and the demographic of the hunter. Thus, this issue is quite complicated despite the fact that cultural representations tend to simplify the situation by leaning on established stereotypes. What perhaps makes this issue even more complicated is that there is another type of animal harm very similar to hunting that evokes little outrage, even though it is responsible for more animal deaths than any other: fishing.

It is estimated that 2.7 trillion fish are killed each year, making them the most-common victims of speciesism globally in terms of numbers (Safina 2018). This is a rough estimate because, unlike mammals, the number of fish slaughtered is usually recorded by mass weight, rather than individual bodies (Cottee 2012: 5–15). As with farming, and in contrast to hunting, the fishing industry has grown significantly over the past hundred years. For example, from 1950 to 1990, consumer demand for fish doubled (Hollander 2003: 56). As demonstrated by the socio-zoological scale, marine mammals are usually offered greater respect and ethical consideration than non-mammal marine life, such as fish and crustaceans. For example, there is a growing demand for dolphin-friendly tuna. This is tuna fish products that did not harm dolphins during the fishing process. Thus, the people that buy this product likely care about dolphin welfare, but they do not have the same respect for tuna fish (Watson 2015). This suggests that it is socially-unacceptable to harm marine mammals, yet socially-acceptable to harm fish. Further to this, and unlike hunting, there are few laws to protect fish from harm (Brown 2015: 3). However, because of oceanic pollution and over-fishing, there have been recent changes in attitudes towards fishing. For example, the "catch and release" fishing method has recently gained popularity. This is when the fisher releases the fish they catch back into the water. The purpose of this is to preserve fish stocks (Rose 2010). However, this practice is arguably unethical as it is likely very traumatizing for the fish involved, even though they mostly survive this process (Rose 2010).

The main reason why fish are subject to speciesist attitudes is likely because humans are unable to empathise with fish suffering in the same way that they can with the suffering of other animals, such as mammals (Hill and Broom 2009: 531–44). There are several reasons why this may be the case. First, it is believed that the appearance and behaviour of fish, such as their scaly skin and lack of vocalizations, stops humans from having the same level of empathy that they do towards species similar to themselves, such as apes and dogs (Elder 2014: 16–29). Humans prefer animals similar to themselves in both appearance and behaviour, such as other mammals. Second, since fish are much smaller than humans and travel in large groups, it is much harder for humans to individualize, and thus anthropomorphise, them (Wadewitz 2011: 425). This leads to the "collapse of compassion" effect. Third, humans rarely experience fish in their natural environments (Brown 2015: 2). As a result, humans are unable to relate to fish as much as they can with animals who share human environments, such as cats. Cumulatively, these three reasons help explain why there is less concern for fish and thus less backlash against fishing as a practice.

Animal rights campaigners have often been accused of ignoring the harms fish experience. For example, one of the most notable marine charities is the Sea Shepherd's Conservation Society (SSCS). The SSCS is an anti-hunting charity that focuses on marine mammals, rather than fish and crustaceans. The majority of the SSCS's operations have been to stop whaling and sealing, rather than fishing (*Sea Shepherd* 2019). However, this may be because the few pro-fish campaigns by animal rights groups have been unsuccessful. For example, in 2009, PETA launched a website which rebranded fish as "sea kittens" in an effort to change public opinions (Newkirk 2009). The fish in the image are notably anthropomorphised and neotenized in a manner similar to how Disney animates animals. However, the fish characters featured in this campaign did not achieve the same level of prevalence as Disney's animal characters frequently do. In fact, this campaign was mocked for being "bizarre" and "idiotic" (*The Daily Telegraph* 2009). This reaction contrasts with the strong, emotive, reaction people often display towards hunting, as demonstrated by the "Cecil effect".

One of the most famous films that features fishing is 1975's *Jaws*. However, this film does not oppose fishing; it supports and justifies it. *Jaws* is about a predatory shark that intentionally kills several humans. The film implies early on that the shark is consciously hunting humans. The film ends with the shark being intentionally killed by an explosion, much to the relief of the surviving human characters. *Jaws* is a strong example of the effect that film can have upon specific animal species. The film is linked with a sharp rise in the numbers of false shark sightings, increased phobias of sharks, and the "*Jaws*-effect". The "*Jaws*-effect" refers to the mass-slaughtering of sharks by fishermen after the release of *Jaws*. This led to a dramatic decrease in shark populations by as much as 90% (Choi 2010). In fact, the backlash against sharks was so severe that Peter Benchley (the book's author) expressed much regret over writing the book and spent the later years of his life campaigning for shark conservation (Donnelly 2015). The attacks have since stopped, but certain species of sharks have not yet recovered their populations (Neff 2015: 114–127). The reaction to *Jaws* demonstrates that when hunting or fishing are depicted as necessary for human survival, it can cause an increase in hunting or fishing in reality.

To conclude Part I of this chapter, it is clear that while hunting and fishing are analogous practices, responses to these practices differ greatly because of speciesist attitudes, cultural representations, and the individual people involved. Hunting is a controversial area of animal studies, yet fishing is probably one of the areas with the least concern, even though it is responsible for more animal deaths than any other form of animal harm. Unlike many other species, the welfare of fish is less-concerning to humans because fish are not individualized, they are un-empathetic, and they are rarely seen in their natural environment. The recent considerations towards fishing (such as the "catch and release" fishing method) have come from a place of environmental concern, rather than because people care about the welfare of fish. In contrast, hunting affects singular members of highly-ranked species that humans are sympathetic towards. As a result, hunting is today vilified in cultural representations, which may be why it has become socially-unacceptable. The only form of hunting that is widely-viewed as socially-acceptable is indigenous hunting, subsistence hunting, or the hunting of villainous animals. These points are further evident with an analysis of WDAS films.

Part II: Data

Please see page 127–129 for a full detailed list of all human-on-animal hunting and fishing in WDAS films.

- Eleven films (20%) feature human-on-animal hunting. Out of the eleven times humans hunt, four instances (36%) result in the definite death of an animal (*Bambi*, *The Fox and the Hound*, *Beauty and the Beast*, and *Brother Bear*). 91% of WDAS's hunters are male. There is only one female hunter (Cruella De Vil), and she is unsuccessful.
- Eight films (14%) feature humans fishing. In 87% of films, the fishers are male. WDAS has only depicted a female fishing once (*Mulan*). Out of the eight times humans are depicted fishing, seven instances result in the definite death of fish (*Pocahontas* does not explicitly depict fish being caught).

Part III: Hunting and Fishing in WDAS Films

As highlighted elsewhere in this book, many of Walt Disney's biographies claim that Walt was a proud animal-lover who often sympathized with the harms animals can face. This attitude was perhaps influenced by two traumatic events that occurred during Walt's early childhood. First, it is well-documented that Walt was traumatized as a young boy after accidently killing an owl:

> It was sitting on the low branch of a tree as I crept up behind it and made a grab. The bird, half-blinded by the daylight, whirled on me and nearly scared me to death. In my terror I stamped on the owl and killed it. I've never forgotten that poor bird, and maybe that has something to do with my liking for animals. (Walt, in: Jackson 2005: 11)

Second, Walt's beloved childhood farm was overrun with wild rabbits. One day, Walt's older brother Roy shot the biggest of these rabbits with an air rifle, and then broke its neck in front of Walt. Walt was apparently distraught by Roy's behaviour and refused to eat the rabbit stew his mother later served that evening (Cartmill 1996: 166–7). These two anecdotes perhaps help explain why hunters, and the unjustified harming of animals generally, have often been presented unfavourably in WDAS films.

From the data presented in Part II, some patterns and similarities are evident with WDAS's portrayal of hunting. First, it is quite notable that the majority of hunting in WDAS films takes place in pre-industrial settings. For example, *The Sword and the Stone*, *Beauty and the Beast*, and *The Princess and the Frog* are all set in the past, i.e. before hunting declined in practice. As highlighted in the previous chapter, this is also true of animal farming. By setting their narratives in the past, WDAS can easily avoid addressing the modern difficulties between humans and animals. For example, by setting their farms in the pre-industrial era, WDAS can avoid addressing the issue of modern megafarms. However, by doing this, WDAS is benefitting from animals by using them to create engaging films, yet they are not benefitting animals in reality because they are ignoring the challenges most animals today experience. Second, all four

WDAS films featuring indigenous cultures (*Pocahontas*, *Mulan*, *Brother Bear*, and *Moana*) include either hunting or fishing, and in two cases both. This is notable because, as highlighted earlier, the hunting and fishing practices of indigenous cultures are the most controversial part of this debate. This will be further discussed in Part IV of this chapter. Third, it is significant that while anthropomorphised animals are sometimes hunted, it is the mostly non-anthropomorphised animals that are killed during hunting (*Bambi* being the notable and very famous exception to this point). Fourth, WDAS does accurately depict that hunting and fishing are male-dominated practices (Cartmill 1996: 233). They have only once depicted a female hunter and female fisher once. However, in the fishing instance, it is Mulan, who is pretending to be male. *Mulan* (1998) is about a female who pretends to be male to save her father from having to enlist in the army. She unsuccessfully fishes as part of her army training. It is implied that her lack of success is because she is female. Fifth, hunters are usually villainous, but not in every instance. For example, in "Peter and the Wolf", it is the hunted wolf that is the villain, not Peter.

WDAS's hunters are usually villainous characters that unjustifiably hunt anthropomorphised animals with weapons. Forbes (2011) claims that there are two types of fictional villains – the repellent and the intriguing – both of which have different narratives, purposes, and meanings (2011: 14). The repellent villains commit worse crimes, which, within the context of animal harm and objectification, usually involve unnecessary suffering and death. Forbes uses the villainous characters in Holocaust-focussed films, such as *Schindler's List* (1993), to exemplify repellent villains, and the types of crimes they commonly commit. However, because of this, films featuring repellent villains are harder to identify with and thus less engaging. This is why repellent villains, such as the hunters in *Bambi*, are much rarer than the intriguing villain, such as someone like Cruella De Vil. In WDAS films, the worst types of direct animal harm (i.e. that which results in death or suffering) are usually committed by faceless or off-screen human characters. The shadowed deer hunters in *Bambi* are one such example of this. As mentioned, this type of villain is rare in WDAS films. In fact, WDAS has on occasion removed this type of villain when adapting external texts. For example, WDAS's 1967 adaptation of Rudyard Kipling's *The Jungle Book* (1893–4) completely removed Buldeo, a prominent human hunter and villain in Kipling's text. Buldeo is a repellent villain that tries to kill several of the jungle animals and Mowgli. Buldeo has been excluded from all of Disney's *The Jungle Book* adaptations so far in favour of more intriguing comical animal villains. Additionally, in WDAS films, the repellent villain is sometimes reformed by the end of a film, usually due to their experiences with the (often anthropomorphised) animal characters. For example, in *The Fox and the Hound*, Amos is introduced as a cruel farmer who hates foxes. However, during the film's climax, Amos's hunting dog Copper protects the hunted fox, Tod, from being shot. This heroic act by Copper appears to change Amos's character for the better. Later, during the film's ending, Amos is depicted with a changed, more-relaxed, outlook towards life. During his last scene, Amos is seen allowing the sweet-natured Widow Tweed to bandage his broken leg, which is an improvement on his previous aggressive and violent character. It is also notable that Amos no longer has his hunting gun in this scene, which had previously been by his side for most of the text.

Forbes' other villain-type, the intriguing villain, is much more common in WDAS films. WDAS often depicts humans who directly harm animals as humorous, overly-dramatic, or cartoonish. This type of character can be seen with Peter from *Make Mine Music* (1946), Gaston in *Beauty and the Beast* (1991), and Clayton in *Tarzan* (1999). Classic Disney animators, Ollie Johnston and Frank Thomas, seemed to acknowledge this character type when they claimed that: "A villainess, even though chilling and dramatic, should have appeal; otherwise, you will not want to watch what she is doing" (Thomas and Johnston 1981: 68). They later added (in a different text) that "The villains we created together at the Disney studio were memorable because they were entertaining" (Johnston and Thomas 1993: 18–19). This demonstrates that WDAS was aware that their villains had to be intriguing if they were to be engaging and memorable. As Chap. 3 will demonstrate, WDAS's most revived villain has been Cruella De Vil, who is undoubtedly an intriguing villain.

As is clear from this chapter's data, there is another type of WDAS hunter that is not depicted as villainous, and that is the justified hunter. Peter from *Make Mine Music* is an example of this character. Peter hunts and catches a wolf, but the wolf he hunts is villainous. It is implied early in the story that the duck (Sonya) has been eaten by the wolf, which is why Peter subsequently hunts the wolf. This immediately establishes the wolf as villainous and Peter as the hero who is trying to save the innocent hunted animals. This is similar to how shark-hunting was justified in *Jaws*. *Jaws* begins with a young woman being killed by the shark, which then justifies the later hunting of the shark. The justified hunter occasionally overlaps with the intriguing villain, but never with the repellent villain. This type of hunter is rare, however. In fact, characters that one would reasonably expect to be depicted as justified hunters, such as Robin Hood (*Robin Hood*) and Mowgli (*The Jungle Book*), do not hunt. For example, in *The Jungle Book*, Mowgli is never seen hunting or eating meat, even though he is raised with a wild wolf pack (Whitley 2008: 104). The context would justify presenting Mowgli as a subsistence hunter, yet WDAS does not.

In reality, hunting is often practiced by groups of men (Flynn 2012: 24–5). This has occasionally been depicted in WDAS films, but usually as background characterization, rather than as part of the main plot (Flynn 2012: 24–5). For example, the deer hunting in *Bambi* (1942) and the bear hunting in *Brother Bear* (2003) are both conducted by groups of men. A key example of this behaviour is in the introductory scene of *Beauty and the Beast*, in which Gaston shoots a bird from the sky that is quickly picked up by his obedient sidekick, Le Fou. Hunting bonds these characters and establishes their masculinity. The bird that Gaston shoots is in the background of the action, non-anthropomorphised, and never mentioned again. Thus, the purpose of this scene is to characterize Gaston and LeFou as toxically-masculine characters, which is indeed how their role in the story continues. WDAS has only ever depicted groups of male hunters; there are no examples of a female group of hunters in WDAS films at all.

WDAS's hunters often have companion animals to help them hunt. These are usually dogs or horses. Such animals are not usually anthropomorphised or individualized even though they co-exist with other individualized and anthropomorphised animals in their diegetic world. For example, in *Bambi*, the hunting dogs that assist the hunters are not anthropomorphised or individualized at all, which contrasts with the individualized, named, and anthropomorphised woodland creatures depicted throughout the film. In several cases, these companion animals die or are seriously injured during their hunts. However, the narratives present the deaths of these animals much less sympathetically than the deaths of individualized animal characters, such as Bambi's mother or Mufasa in *The Lion King*. For example, after the hunting dogs in *Bambi* fall off a cliff, presumably to their deaths, there is no solemn music or pained reaction from the other animals. Therefore, it seems that the injury or death of an animal that harms other animals is depicted as justifiable. Similarly, as demonstrated earlier with *Jaws*, cultural depictions commonly imply that it is acceptable to hunt and kill animals that harm humans or other animals. The one exception to these points is *The Fox and the Hound*, in which this exception to the norm forms the main storyline.

In WDAS films, anthropomorphised hunted animals usually survive being prey. In fact, even some anthropomorphised fish have survived being fished, which is surprising given how WDAS has depicted fishing generally. However, the fact that anthropomorphised animals survive routine animal harm, whereas non-anthropomorphised animal characters do not, is anthropocentric. It implies that only animals that behave in human-like ways are worthy of avoiding harm and death. To illustrate, the deaths of the non-anthropomorphised, non-neotenous, hunting dogs in *Bambi* is presented in a justified manner because of the animalistic aggression they demonstrated previously towards other animals. In contrast, the deaths of anthropomorphised, neotenous, individualized animals, such as Bambi's mother, are reflected upon in the narrative in a sympathetic manner.

WDAS's most famous film centred around hunting is undoubtedly 1942's *Bambi*, a film so emotionally-charged, it has been cited as a catalyst for the decline in the social-acceptance of hunting (Lutts 1992: 160). *Bambi* was adapted from *Bambi, A Life in the Woods* (1923) by Felix Salten. Unlike Walt, Salten was a hunter and even owned his own hunting preserve (Cartmill 1996: 163). This is noteworthy because *Bambi, A Life in the* Woods is critical of hunters and sympathetic towards hunted animals (Cartmill 1996: 163). Salten's novel was criticized for its realistic graphic violence. For example, in Salten's text, a ferret kills a mouse, crows attack a baby hare, and Bambi is shot in the shoulder (Cartmill

1996: 163–4). Much of this violence was removed or attenuated during WDAS's adaptation process. Yet despite removing many of the darker elements of the text, the WDAS adaptation did emphasize realism. During the making of *Bambi*, the animators benefitted from drawing lessons, trips to the zoo, and live and dead deer. This allowed them to accurately design the animal species depicted (Riffel 2012: 13).[5]

WDAS's *Bambi* depicts an almost-perfect harmonious woodland life that is carelessly disrupted by human hunters. The film follows various woodland animals from infancy to adulthood who quickly learn to fear "man", i.e. hunters. The different animal species in the film respect and care for each other and are united against their understandable fear of humans. The woodland creatures only seem to eat vegetation, such as flowers, and they are never shown eating meat. The only naturally carnivorous animals in WDAS's version are an owl and a skunk, yet neither are depicted as hunting or eating other animals (Hastings 1996: 53–9). This is in contrast to Salten's original text, which contained several instances of fatal animal-on-animal hunting (Hastings 1996: 53–9).

The death of Bambi's mother was a fully-storyboarded scene, but it was not included in the film's final edit (Beiman 2007: 281). Instead, the film shows what happens during hunting, and its repercussions. Midway through the film, Bambi and his mother are chased by hunters. Bambi runs ahead of his mother and safely manages to hide in some bushes. Once Bambi is safe, a loud gunshot is heard, but not shown. Bambi is then shown naively calling and looking for his mother, clearly unaware of what the gunshot indicated. The off-screen gunshot a few seconds earlier and solemn music imply that Bambi's mother has been shot and killed. However, the body of Bambi's mother is never depicted. Her death is soon confirmed by the re-appearance of Bambi's father, The Great Prince of the Forest. The death of Bambi's mother is vital to make the film's anti-hunting message work. This scene focusses on the unnecessary loss of an infant's mother, a situation that most people can empathise with (Hastings 1996: 53–9). Thus, this moment demonstrates why hunting is immoral:

---

[5] While these production methods were innovative at the time, they were expensive, which is why WDAS never repeated this with any other WDAS films. *Bambi* took six years to make and made less revenue than expected, but this was partly due to World War Two (Pallant 2010a: 350).

it can result in the death of animals, and in doing so, can leave other animals parentless.

Even though *Bambi* is most famous for its emotional hunting scenes, these comprise just a small portion of the film (Whitley 2008: 66). In fact, the hunters only appear thrice. While the animals in *Bambi* are rendered in great detail, the human characters are not; they are never fully-shown onscreen, nor do they speak (Hastings 1996: 53–9). They exist as shadows and through the sound of gunshots. Even when the human camp is shown, there are no hunters visible. As noted earlier, Forbes (2011) argues that villains fall into two categories: intriguing and repellent. The hunters in *Bambi* are the repellent type. This repellent character is aided by their lack of physical appearance. Additionally, by not being developed characters, there is little opportunity for the narrative to convey a reason for their hunting. In "Peter and the Wolf", Peter's hunting is justified through the wolf's earlier villainy. This is not the case in *Bambi*; the hunters' motives remain mysterious, and so it appears as if they have no justifiable motive for their actions.

Bambi has often been criticized by pro-hunting groups for its depiction of hunters as irresponsible. The film's shadowy hunters violate several rules of modern ethical hunting practices, such as being careless with their campfire, hunting out of season, and shooting animals carelessly (Hastings 1996: 53–9). Upon the film's release, American hunters argued that this carelessness did not represent the majority of modern hunters (Hastings 1996: 53–9). For example, in the 1942 edition of the pro-hunting magazine *Outdoor Life*, the editor Raymond Brown claimed that the film was: "The worst insult ever offered in any form to American sportsmen" (Cartmill 1996: 178). Brown's concern that the film might tarnish hunting's reputation was not ill-founded as hunting significantly declined as a practice after the film's release (Hastings 1996: 53–9). Indeed, the film's anti-hunting message is still used today. In 2018, a deer poacher in America was ordered to watch *Bambi* once a month during his year-long jail sentence for killing hundreds of animals illegally (*The Guardian* 2018). After *Bambi*, WDAS depicted several other unethical and inconsiderate hunters, such as Amos Slade in *The Fox and the Hound* (1981) and Clayton in *Tarzan* (1999). For example, in *Tarzan* (1999), Clayton is dramatically introduced to the film with the sound of several loud gunshots. Then, he carelessly chops down parts of the jungle with a machete, desperate to find some gorillas. Furthermore, Clayton frequently shoots his shotgun randomly, without any care for the animals or environment around him. This demonstrates that WDAS is committed to their depiction of hunters as both unethical and irresponsible. This demonstrates that WDAS evidently did not uphold the complaints real hunters had about the film.

It has been noted that children's media exhibits an overwhelming opposition to hunting, which seems to have begun in the children's literature of the eighteenth century and continues to the present day (Hastings 1996: 53–9). For this reason, some researchers have claimed that *Bambi* should not be given sole credit for changing public opinion on hunting, as this was actually the work of many anti-hunting texts (Hastings 1996: 53–9). Another film suggested to have affected public attitudes towards hunting is 1978's *Watership Down*. *Watership Down* depicts animal-on-animal hunting and human-on-animal hunting; however, it does so in a much more graphic way than WDAS ever has. At the beginning of the story, one of the female rabbits (Violet) is hunted and killed by a hawk. Later, another female rabbit (Hazel) is shot by a farmer. Both of these moments occur onscreen and involve explicit bloodshed.[6] These visual elements contrast with WDAS's depictions of hunting, which usually occur off-screen and are implied, rather than literally depicted. However, it seems that this lack of onscreen violence may have worked in WDAS's favour. *Watership Down* subsequently became infamous for these bloody scenes rather than famous for its artistic merits (Hoad 2014). Perhaps for this reason, *Bambi* and *Watership Down* have left vastly different legacies. For example, *Bambi* merchandise is still widely-sold today, suggesting that the characters are seen affectionately, despite the story's darker tones.[7]

In contrast to WDAS's hunters, WDAS's fishers are never portrayed as villains. In WDAS films, fish are usually non-anthropomorphised background objects rather than individualized animal characters. For

[6] Upon its release, the BBFC received many complaints about *Watership Down* due to its "U" certification (*BBFC* 2010). A "U" certification means that the film is suitable for children, which many felt was not the case with *Watership Down* (for example: Barnes 2016).

[7] For example, Disney's UK shops still stock various types of *Bambi* merchandise, such as clothing, soft toys, and crockery (*Shop Disney* 2019a).

example, in *Fun and Fancy Free*, Bongo the circus bear juggles a fish in a goldfish bowl amongst other objects as part of his circus act. Similarly, in *Beauty and the Beast*, a non-anthropomorphised goldfish lives inside an anthropomorphised clock. Thus, WDAS's fish characters are often depicted as nothing more than background objects rather than living, sentient, animals. There are believed to be over 32,000 species of fish (Brown 2015: 1). However, only twenty-one distinct fish species have been depicted in WDAS films. Additionally, this text's data produced a category of ambiguous fish (fish without a clear species). Ambiguous fish can be seen in nineteen WDAS films, which is more than a third of WDAS films (1937–2016). Additionally, this is more than the amount of times any clear species of fish is depicted. Therefore, WDAS is depicting ambiguous fish more often than any clear species of fish. There is no equivalent "ambiguous" category for mammals. This further highlights that WDAS's fish are often undetailed, and without a clear character or species. Furthermore, the fish that do exist in WDAS films are usually not anthropomorphised or named. In fact, WDAS has never characterized a fish as a protagonist or antagonist.

When the practice of fishing is shown, it is often un-sympathetic towards the fish. During "Piano Concerto No. 2", the fourth segment of *Fantasia 2000*, an anthropomorphised toy soldier finds himself in the sea after fighting with another toy in his home. The toy escapes the sea after being caught in a large fishing net amongst hundreds of non-anthropomorphised fish. Because the toy is anthropomorphised and individualized, and the fish are not, the narrative encourages more sympathy for the toy, leaving the fish as background objects. The fish and the toy soldier are boxed up and sold, which allows the toy soldier to find his way home serendipitously. Therefore, the lives and welfare of many fish are depicted as less-worthy of consideration than one toy soldier.

To conclude Part III, it is evident that WDAS has often criticized hunting, most notably with *Bambi*. Most of WDAS's hunters have been villainous characters acting maliciously and carelessly. There are various types of hunters in WDAS films, such as grouped, the repellent, the intriguing, and the justified. In contrast, WDAS has shown little interest in criticizing fishing. Fish are rarely individualized or anthropomorphised in WDAS films. Additionally, fishing as a practice is usually portrayed as socially-acceptable. Unlike other forms of animal harm such as farming, fishing is not even romanticized, suggesting that there is nothing upsetting or unethical about this practice. The next section of this chapter will explore how hunting and fishing are depicted in 2003's *Brother Bear*. This is a WDAS film that reflects and reinforces the wider inconsistent speciesist and socially-acceptable attitudes towards both hunting and fishing.

Part IV: Hunting, Fishing, and *Brother Bear* (2003)

It may seem odd that *Bambi* is not this chapter's case study given that it is undoubtedly WDAS's most famous anti-hunting film. However, as is clear from Part III of this chapter, *Bambi* has already received intense academic attention. Furthermore, *Bambi* does not question and explore the motives of hunters. Additionally, *Bambi* only demonstrates how WDAS has depicted hunting. It does not explore fishing, which raises similar ethical concerns to hunting. Therefore, this chapter will instead conclude by studying the depictions of hunting and fishing in *Brother Bear*, a Neo-Disney WDAS film that has not received much academic attention to-date.

In *Brother Bear*, an Alaskan Inuit hunter (Kenai) is transformed into an anthropomorphised bear after maliciously hunting and killing a non-anthropomorphised bear. This transformation drastically reverses Kenai's opinion on hunting. As a bear, Kenai is himself hunted by humans, leading him to understand why animals fear hunters. However, despite the film's anti-hunting message, *Brother Bear* exhibits speciesist bias because it only focusses on the cruelty of harming mammals and birds. Other animal species, such as fish and insects, are directly objectified and harmed in the film. This makes the film's seemingly pro-animal message problematic.

As highlighted in Part I, indigenous hunting is a contentious issue and not often criticized in the same way that hunting practiced by Anglo-Americans is. Therefore, it is perhaps surprising that WDAS chose to produce an anti-hunting story with characters based upon indigenous people, especially given WDAS's own problematic history with depictions of race and indigenous people.[8] However, while WDAS's past portrayals of indigenous communities have been criticized, it was not for how they portrayed the use of animals within these cultures. In fact, WDAS has usually romanticized the way that indigenous societies use animals, rather than criticized them. For example, in *Pocahontas*, it is implied that the Native Americans have an affinity with nature that the settlers do not. The Native Americans are depicted as an ethical organic farming and fishing community, whereas the British settlers are presented as merciless hunters with little understanding of nature (Whitley 2008: 85). For example, Pocahontas stops John Smith from shooting a bear on-sight during the "Colours of the Wind" montage (Whitley 2008: 85). After stopping Smith, Pocahontas picks up a bear cub of the larger bear Smith attempted to shoot, seemingly educating Smith on the local wildlife (Whitley 2008: 87). However, the message here is somewhat confusing; Pocahontas teaches Smith not to hunt, but she then metaphorically objectifies the bears by playing with them as if they are pets (Whitley 2008: 87). The "Colours of the Wind" song that plays over this moment implies that Pocahontas's actions are the ones that are more natural and moral. Yet by picking up the bear cub, Pocahontas (and the narrative) ignores the instinctive murderous response of the mother bear (Whitley 2008: 87). Thus, the hunting instincts of wild animals and the behaviour of the Native Americans are romanticized. Some of the Native Americans are depicted with bows and arrows, which implies that they do hunt animals; however, only John Smith is depicted hunting and as treating animals badly. WDAS seems to be implying here that the Native American's treatment of animals is more ethical because they live alongside them. This may be because the indigenous people have a legitimate claim over the land they are on, which Smith does not. This romanticization is troubling given that colonists traditionally labelled indigenous people as animalistic or savage, which depictions like this seem to support by presenting Native Americans as being harmoniously connected to nature (Mechling

[8] For example, a history of how WDAS has problematically depicted Native Americans can be found in: Prajna Parasher 'Mapping the Imaginary: The Neverland of Disney's Indians' (Parasher 2013).

2004: 69). Furthermore, *Pocahontas* attempts to present the Native Americans as non-predatory near-vegetarians in a perfect world that balances nature (Whitley 2008: 85). However, Native Americans are not traditionally pescatarian, so this is a misleading depiction that likely exists only to romanticize the Native Americans and further the stereotype that they have an affinity with animals. A similar criticism can be applied to *Brother Bear*, which also romanticizes the Inuit-animal relationship. In *Brother Bear*, the Inuit characters have an affinity with nature. However, Kenai breaks this affinity by hunting a bear out of malice rather than necessity. As in *Bambi*, the different non-human animal species in *Brother Bear* live harmoniously with each other, with man as their only enemy. There are no villainous or predatory animals, nor are any animals depicted eating meat (with the notable exception of fish).

Kenai, the protagonist of *Brother Bear*, begins the narrative as disrespectful towards animals, which is in contrast to the other members of his tribe. For example, during the film's opening montage, he rides a distressed mammoth for his own amusement. It is soon mentioned that Kenai will be receiving his totem from the tribal shaman later that day, signifying that he has come of age. Kenai tells some children that he expects a sabre tooth tiger as his totem; thus, he shows a preference for a higher-order carnivorous animal. However, much to his disappointment, Kenai is given a bear instead. Soon after Kenai receives his totem, one of his brothers (Sitka) dies after falling from ice during a bear hunt. This leads Kenai to blaming the bear for the tragedy and vowing revenge. Kenai's other brother (Denahi) warns Kenai that his abrupt reaction is unnecessary, unspiritual, and unnatural. As evidenced in Part I, it was believed in the past that respectful hunters were better hunters, which may be what Denahi's belief is based upon. However, Kenai hunts and kills the bear anyway. The bear's death leads to a spiritual switch between Kenai and the bear's body. It later transpires that the bear had a cub, which is now orphaned because of Kenai. At first, Kenai does not understand that he is a bear, or why many other animals are scared of him. Kenai decides to head towards the Northern Lights, where he believes he will be able to transform back into human form. Kenai is helped along his journey by Koda (the bear cub whom he orphaned).[9] However, Koda and Kenai's journey becomes dangerous after they are tracked by Denahi, Sitka's brother. Denahi (who is still human) is angry that both Kenai and Sitka were killed by the same bear, so he hunts the bear, which unbeknownst to him is now Kenai. This allows Kenai to see how terrifying hunting is for bears and other animals, causing him to reverse his opinion on hunting.

Once Kenai and Koda arrive at the "salmon run" (which is in the same direction as the Northern Lights), Kenai realizes that Koda's mother is dead, and that Kenai was the hunter who killed her. During this scene, Koda tells the story of how his mother was hunted, but it is clear that Koda does not know that his mother is dead; he believes that she is missing. While this flashback is similar in narrative structure to the death of Bambi's mother in *Bambi*, it does not hold the same emotional power. This is partly because by this point, the narrative has encouraged sympathy for Kenai's situation. Kenai killed the bear because he was grieving his brother's death, as such he is able to show regret in hindsight. In *Bambi*, however, the hunters' intentions are never explained, suggesting a lack of remorse and regret. Additionally, in *Brother Bear*, the hunt is much fairer since the hunters do not have guns and are smaller than the bear. In *Bambi*, the animals can only run away; they have no chance to fight back against the hunters, making the situation unfair in contrast. Additionally, Koda's mother is not anthropomorphised, which Bambi's mother was.

While the anti-hunting message of the film is clear, similar forms of animal harm are not criticized; in fact, some are celebrated. The narrative drives towards a fairly complicated dissection of why hunting might be problematic, then displays a similar practice (fishing) as being completely acceptable. The film opens with the three (human) brothers bonding through fishing. The numerous non-anthropomorphised fish that they catch are kept in a leather fishing net and brought back to their camp. Kenai is then shown emptying the bag of dead fish into a basket in front of some children who show no disgust over the situation. The children

[9] The body of Koda's mother is the body that Kenai transforms into. However, the fact that Koda's mother was female and Kenai is male is not elaborated on in the film. Furthermore, Koda does not appear to recognise his mother as Kenai. Thus, even though Kenai is depicted as transforming into the bear he killed, there are plot holes within this narrative.

hold the basket for Kenai and chat to him as he empties the fish into it. This lack of disgust highlights the practice's social acceptance within the tribe. Later in the film, during Kenai and Koda's journey to the Northern Lights, Kenai and Koda participate in the bears' annual "salmon run". Upon arrival, they see a sleuth of bears fishing salmon as the upbeat song "Welcome" plays over them. Ironically, this song celebrates the beauty of nature, even though the scene depicts bears killing and eating numerous live fish raw. For example, some of the lyrics are: "This has to be the most beautiful, the most peaceful place I've ever been to. It's nothing like I've never seen before". This is a harmonious and cheerful scene that celebrates the friendship of the bears, and the moral lessons learnt by Kenai. The salmon are not anthropomorphised, and there is no blood or distress from them. This characterizes them as objects rather than sentient animals. Thus, the narrative does not encourage viewers to reflect upon the deaths of these fish. Later in this scene, the bears pass around a decapitated fish as they take turns telling their stories from the year. Again, fish are clearly presented as objects here rather than animals. However, this speciesism towards fish is somewhat acknowledged at the end of the film, albeit in a comical manner. After some of the end credits, Koda addresses the audience and tells them that: "In accordance with all federal and state law regulations, no fish were harmed during the making of the film". This clearly mimics the American Humane Association's end-of-film "No animals were harmed..." message that accompanies live-action films which have used animals.[10] As Koda speaks, a bear can be seen in the background chasing an anthropomorphised salmon. The salmon leaps from the water and screams in a human-like manner as it is chased. This is the only anthropomorphised fish in the entire film, and it is part of a joke about animal harm. Additionally, this one anthropomorphised fish is not caught and thus does not die, which is in contrast with the numerous non-anthropomorphised fish that do die unceremoniously in the main narrative. This scene also reinforces the point that anthropomorphised animal characters experience less harm than non-anthropomorphised ones in WDAS films.

[10] The AHA will be further discussed in Chap. 5.

The fact that WDAS offers much more respect to anthropomorphised animals is evident with other animal characters in the film too. In *Brother Bear*, none of the animals are anthropomorphised until Kenai metamorphoses into a bear. Yet even after Kenai's metamorphosis, some animals remain non-anthropomorphised, notably the salmon, but also the insects. For example, the fleas on the moose are not anthropomorphised, but the moose that they live on are. The moose can speak English, which provides comic relief throughout the film. The lack of anthropomorphism given to the insect and fish characters is consistent with how WDAS has depicted lower-order species generally; they are rarely anthropomorphised, nor are they ever primary characters.

To conclude Part IV, it is clear that *Brother Bear* reinforces many of WDAS's anti-hunting notions, but it also reinforces many of their speciesist attitudes too. The film clearly depicts hunting as an unfair and uncivilized practice, yet it also presents fishing as completely acceptable, as long as the fish are non-anthropomorphised. Thus, *Brother Bear* is another film that highlights the importance of anthropomorphism in WDAS films; anthropomorphised animal characters evidently experience far less harm than non-anthropomorphised ones. Furthermore, the film justifies the hunting practices of indigenous people by allowing Kenai to show remorse for his actions in hindsight, which WDAS does not do for other groups, such as toxically-masculine Anglo-American men, like Percival McLeach (*The Rescuers Down Under*) or John Smith (*Pocahontas*). This highlights WDAS's bias on certain issues. They are evidently only comfortable criticizing practices and groups of people that are socially-acceptable to do so.

Conclusion

WDAS's history spans across the sharp decline of hunting in the Anglo-American world. WDAS can take a small amount of the credit for this decline with their unflattering portrayals of hunting and hunters, particularly with *Bambi*. However, in WDAS's lifetime, fishing has risen towards dangerous and uncontrollable levels, which they have shown little concern for. There are a few reasons for this. Hunting and fishing are analogous practices; however, they involve different species and numbers of animals as well as demographics of humans, and all of these factors significantly affect how the public react towards animal welfare issues. In WDAS films, fish are only occasionally spared from fishing, but only when they are anthropomorphised and individualized, which is rarely. In contrast, the ethics of hunting forms the main plot line of several WDAS films, such as *Bambi*, *The Fox and the Hound*, and *Brother Bear*.

The next chapter of this book will consider how WDAS has presented clothing and other products made from the bodies of animals. The findings of this chapter follow through into the next argument: the products of high-order and individualized species (such as dogs) are deemed to be unacceptable, yet products made from fish (such as shell jewellery) are acceptable. Moreover, the demographics of the consumer affect the social-acceptance of the issue. These ideas are, again, reinforced by WDAS films, as the next chapter will demonstrate.

3

Clothing and Other Objects Made from Animals

In 2010, the pop star Lady Gaga famously, or perhaps infamously, wore a dress made of raw beef during a red-carpet appearance (Baron 2016). This "meat dress" attracted much criticism from both the public and animal rights groups (for example: Newkirk 2010). However, the outrage caused by this dress is inconsistent when compared with other attitudes expressed towards Gaga's clothing. Lady Gaga appears to frequently wear leather, a material produced from the same species as her controversial "meat dress" was (for example: Heching 2020). Yet when Gaga wears leather, she attracts almost no criticism, outrage, or attention. It is as if the ethics of wearing meat and leather are separate moral issues, despite both materials originating from the same species and being utilized in similar ways. The public's distaste for Gaga's "meat dress" demonstrates a common logical inconsistency towards clothing made from animal products. This inconsistent reaction is further evident through the common reactions to other non-perishable products made from animals' bodies, such as fur, leather, shells, and so forth.

This chapter will study how WDAS has depicted clothing and other objects made from animals' bodies, such as fur, leather, shells, and feathers. It is clear that while fur has become socially-unacceptable, leather,

R. R. Stanton, *The Disneyfication of Animals*, The Palgrave Macmillan Animal Ethics Series, https://doi.org/10.1007/978-3-030-49316-5_3

shells, and feathers are widely seen as acceptable. This chapter will argue that WDAS and Disney are selective with their criticism of products made from animals' bodies. Additionally, like farming, hunting, and fishing, such criticism is contingent on the species involved as well as the demographics of the consumer. Part I of this chapter will explore the relevant history and discourses surrounding clothing and other objects produced from animals' bodies. Part II will provide data that documents how often these products have been depicted in WDAS films. Then, Part III will examine how WDAS has depicted fur, compared with how they have depicted other clothing and objects, such as leather and feathers. Finally, Part IV will look at WDAS's most famous film about the ethics of producing clothing and other objects from animals: *One Hundred and One Dalmatians* (1961).[1]

Part I: When Animals Become Objects

Fur is believed to be one of the earliest materials used for human clothing, and it was one of the first ways that humans utilized animal bodies (Roth 1997: 354). Originally, fur provided a practical purpose for humans: warmth. However, today, in the Anglo-American world, fur is usually worn on the outer-part of the clothing as a fashion item (Mahe 2011). Historically, humans produced fur clothing from many different mammals, but today, the majority of fur used comes from rodents, such as mink and chinchilla (*Fur Free Alliance* 2018). As with food farming, fur farming was industrialized at the beginning of the twentieth century (Roth 1997: 354). Today, PETA claims that 85% of fur comes from fur farms. These farms usually house thousands of animals with little concern for individual animal welfare (*PETA* 2019n). However, unlike food farming, there has been a significant backlash against fur farming, especially in the Anglo-American world. Moreover, unlike many other backlashes against animal objectification, anti-fur campaigns have successfully led to

[1] Some sections of this chapter are taken from an earlier article written by the same author. That article is due to be published as a chapter in an upcoming book about the ethics of fur. The book is being published through the Palgrave Macmillan Animal Ethics Series (*Palgrave Macmillan* 2019).

widespread changes in law and public opinion as this chapter will demonstrate.

As with fur, humans have been producing and using leather for as long as they have been hunting animals for food (*Moore and Giles* 2018). Leather is renowned worldwide for its durability and comfort, making it much more practical, and thus more widely-used, than fur has been (*Moore and Giles* 2018). For example, throughout human history, humans have used leather to build shelters, make clothing, footwear, buckets, shrouds, and so forth (*Moore and Giles* 2018). As with some other industries that objectify animals, such as the dairy industry, the leather industry has successfully convinced consumers that leather is a sustainable product (*Vegan Life Magazine* 2017). For example, leather is often defended because it has been successfully marketed as a "by-product" of the meat industry (Siegle 2016). This is an argument that the fur industry cannot use because the animals that are used to make fur clothing, such as mink, are not usually consumed. Critics have responded to the "by-product" argument by claiming that leather is a subsidy rather than by-product (*The Guardian* 2008). This is because animal skins are actually the most profitable part of farmed animals (*Vegan Life Magazine* 2017). In fact, the leather industry is worth billions of dollars annually, clearly making it much more than just a by-product (*The Guardian* 2008). In 2016, it was estimated that around 290 million cows die every year to make leather, most of which live on factory farms (Siegle 2016). This figure is predicted to rise to 430 million by 2025 in order to keep up with the growing consumer demand for this material (Siegle 2016). Like the fur industry, the leather industry is responding to the growing changes in consumer opinions by providing more sustainable options, such as pineapple leather (Siegle 2016). However, unlike fur, the current backlash towards leather is rooted in its negative effects on the environment – methane and greenhouse gas produced by livestock – rather than concerns over the welfare of the animals involved (Mosley 2014; Siegle 2016).

Within critical animal studies discourse, the two most-commonly discussed clothing materials made from animals seem to be fur and leather. However, there are several other materials produced from animals' bodies that are regularly used by humans, such as shells, pearls, wool, silk, and feathers (*PETA* 2019n). The animal rights movement has generally campaigned less against these products. The main reason for this is speciesism. For example, shells come from molluscs are not even considered to be an animal by many (Singer 1990: 174; MacClellan 2013: 58). Additionally, unlike fur and leather, pearls, wool, and feathers can be taken from animals without harming or killing them. However, these products are mostly produced in factory farms, meaning that there is a high chance that the animals involved live caged lives and are killed when no longer useful (*Farm Sanctuary* 2018). The production of shells and silk requires the animal to die, but the animals involved (shellfish and silkworms) score so lowly on the socio-zoological scale that their death is not a concern to most people. Because fur and leather are focused on more frequently than other products, this chapter will now question why they are responded to so differently.

Celebrated fashion designer Karl Lagerfeld controversially claimed that "In a meat-eating world, wearing leather for shoes and clothes and even handbags, the discussion of fur is childish" (Adams 2009). By "childish", Lagerfeld is implying that the public's reaction to the fur industry is undercut by a lack of critical reflection on other ways of objectifying animals, such as the production of leather and wool. Lagerfeld's point seems to be affirmed by the ways these products are depicted in Disney texts and represented in culture more broadly. Alongside hunting, the social-acceptance of fur production has sharply dropped since it stopped being necessary for human survival. In fact, fur farms are today banned in many Anglo-American countries. For example, in 2000, the UK proudly banned fur farms ahead of EU legislation (Brown 2001b). This decision clearly reflected public attitude as a 2011 estimate found that 95% of British people opposed the wearing of fur (McVeigh 2014). However, the UK has over eight hundred megafarms, which attract little criticism (Wasley et al. 2017). This demonstrates that different uses of animals are perceived in disparate ways. Thus, the UK seems to only oppose specific types of animal harm and objectification. In fact, the same 2011 survey that found that 95% of British people oppose fur found that just 2% of British people opposed using leather (McVeigh 2014). As highlighted earlier, leather is widely-used in the Anglo-American world, yet it faces very little criticism in comparison to fur. Leather and fur products are produced in similar ways, yet the former rarely evokes the same sympathetic and passionate reactions elicited by the latter. This contradiction can also be applied to the use of feathers, silk, pearls, wool, and shells. It seems clear from both the law and public attitudes that the production of fur is socially-unacceptable, whereas other products made from animals are permissible. This disparity in social-acceptance is clearly about more than just animal welfare.

One difference between fur and other clothing made from animals is the cost. Modern fur products are quite expensive and thus out of most people's price range. For example, designer fur coats generally cost thousands of pounds, which is a prohibitive price for many (Karlson 2013). In fact, one of the few department stores in the UK that still stocks fur clothing is Harrods, a shop famous for its high-cost products (*Harrods* 2018). In contrast, leather, wool, and so forth are usually affordable and available to purchase widely (for example: *Debenhams* 2019). Therefore, these products attract different demographics of customers. As will be highlighted in Part III, this is accurately reflected in WDAS through the types of characters that often wear fur and leather. For example, in WDAS films set in modern narratives, fur is often worn by wealthy women, such as Ms. Bianca (*The Rescuers*) and Cruella (*Dalmatians*). However, leather appears to be often worn by less-wealthy characters, such as Amos (*The Fox and the Hound*). As the previous chapter demonstrated, ways of using or harming animals that are unaffordable to most people, such as trophy hunting, are usually socially-unacceptable. In contrast, ways of using animals that are affordable, such as wearing leather and practicing fishing, are usually socially-acceptable. This suggests that the widespread distaste towards fur is rooted in an underlying anger over wealth disparity.

Another difference is that fur and leather are worn by different demographics. Fur is often advertised at, and thus mostly worn by, wealthy women. As a result, the hatred people exhibit towards fur could stem from a hatred towards rich women (Betts 2012). Relating to this, it has been found that people typically judge crimes committed by females more harshly than they do crimes committed by males (Kennedy 2018). This is believed to be because of society's expectations of women as more nurturing than men (Kennedy 2018). Perhaps because of this expectation, products predominantly used by women that involve animal harm during production are criticized more often than other products. For example, cosmetics (that have been tested on animals) and fur clothing appear to be judged harshly, which has led to many campaigns and legal changes towards these products. For example, since 2013 it has been illegal to sell cosmetics tested on animals in states in the European Union (*RSPCA* 2019a). However, similar products, such as cleaning products, can still be tested on animals and sold in countries such as the UK (Dalton 2019). This suggests that products aimed at women are held to higher standards of animal welfare than products aimed at everyone.

Additionally, the appearance of fur may also contribute towards the public's opposition towards it. Clothing made from fur usually has the same appearance as the species it came from. Thus, another reason why people object to fur clothing is for the same reason that they objected to Gaga's "meat dress": its appearance is redolent of a dead animal. As highlighted in Chap. 1, animal farming is only socially-acceptable because it is attenuated. Leather does not look like the species it was produced from, which is why it is acceptable, yet Gaga's "meat dress" was not. Feather products also look like the animal they came from, but, unlike leather and fur, a bird does not have to be killed to produce feathers, which likely makes it more acceptable. Dairy is more socially-acceptable than meat for the same reason (as dairy cows do not need to be killed to produce milk). Shells also look like the animal they came from, but since they are produced from molluscs, an animal that scores very low on the socio-zoological scale and is not even considered an animal by many, their welfare is not a concern to most humans (MacClellan 2013: 58).

However, the main difference between fur products and other products made from animals is, of course, the species they come from. Anti-fur campaigns suggest that fur usually comes from neotenous fluffy animals that score highly on the socio-zoological scale, such as puppies and seals. As highlighted earlier, this image is false since most fur produced today actually comes from rodents (*Fur Free Alliance* 2018). In contrast, leather comes from livestock, such as cows, which score lower on the socio-zoological scale. Thus, speciesism explains why the production of fur is no longer socially-acceptable. Species that score highly on the socio-zoological scale are often mammals with plentiful body hair, i.e. fluffy animals. It is often these animals whose mistreatment is not socially-acceptable, as is the case with the puppies in *Dalmatians*, for example.

Fur is a neotenous attribute – i.e. excessively furry animals are younger-looking – because baby mammals and birds, such as chicks and puppies, often have much more hair than older animals (Gould 1977).

Fur is also separated from leather and other objects made from animals by the "collapse of compassion" effect and anthropomorphism. The species that the public believe fur comes from, such as dogs, are often individualized and anthropomorphised through pet ownership and the like. Because of this individualization, people typically exhibit greater compassion towards the plight of animals farmed for fur. Other products, such as leather and feathers, are produced from species that are less likely to be anthropomorphised or individualized, such as cattle and birds. Additionally, since these species of animals are not usually kept as pets or used for entertainment, the public has fewer opportunities to individualize them. Thus, the "collapse of compassion" effect occurs, and humans are significantly less-likely to feel concern.

As with farming, hunting, and fishing, cultural representations seem to have influenced how people view fur, leather, and other materials made from animals. As a result, cultural representations are often credited for fur's sharp decline in sales and social acceptance over the past hundred years (O'Connor 2018). Today, fur is widely depicted as unacceptable in cultural representations, even when necessary to the context. For example, *Game of Thrones* (2011–2019) faced much criticism for using real furs as part of their character costumes even though fur clothing was relevant to the show's context (Boydell 2016). The show responded by claiming that the furs used were mostly sourced from vintage markets, rather than purchased from fur retailers (Boydell 2016). This example demonstrates that the entertainment industry is aware of the negative connotations of using fur products. *Game of Thrones* seem to have predicted that their use of fur would be questioned, which is likely why they purchased their furs second-hand rather than new.

In 1994, PETA launched one of their most successful campaigns, in which five supermodels (Emma Sjoberg, Tatiana Patitz, Heather Stewart Whyte, Fabienne Terwinghe, and Naomi Campbell) declared that "We'd rather go naked than wear fur" (Bekhechi 2010). After this campaign, fur became dramatically less fashionable (McVeigh 2014). For example, soon after the advertisement's release, many fur retailers, such as Selfridges, refused to stock it (McVeigh 2014). Unlike many of PETA's campaigns, the "We'd rather go naked…" campaign was not bloody or graphic, instead it simply featured five prolific supermodels naked. Its appeal was its nudity. This campaign has been revived many times with various naked celebrities opposing the use of fur. PETA's naked campaigns tend to be much more influential than their graphic campaigns (Bekhechi 2010). For example, in 2014, PETA released a video titled *Hell for Leather*. This grim footage followed the final hours of a caravan of mistreated cattle travelling in-between India and Bangladesh. After the cattle are skinned alive in front of each other, their skins are processed by child workers (Siegle 2016). As of February 17th, 2019, ten years after the film was released on YouTube, it has accrued fewer than 9000 views. Thus, its potential for impact is minimal compared to PETA's iconic "naked fur" campaign. Furthermore, many of *PETA*'s anti-leather campaigns have been bloody or depicted mistreatment, which may be why they have been less-engaging and thus had less impact (Atkins-Sayre 2010: 309–28). As discussed in Chap. 1, when realistic animal harm is depicted in cultural representations, such as film, it becomes notorious for doing so. Moreover, these types of images rarely result in mainstream success. However, cultural representations that challenge animal harm without being gory and distressing, such as PETA's "We'd rather go naked…" campaign and films such as *Babe* (1995), are evidently far more engaging and thus usually more successful.

To conclude Part I of this chapter, it is clear that, as with other forms of animal objectification, discussions surrounding products made from animals, such as fur and leather, are divided by speciesist attitudes, which cultural representations have helped to sustain. Additionally, fur clothing has been further vilified because of the people who wear it (wealthy western women), its high cost, and its animal-like appearance, which have cumulatively led to it being one of the most opposed areas of animal objectification.

Part II: Data

Please see pages 129–131 of the appendixes for a full list of all depictions of fur, leather, feathers, and shells in the fifty-six WDAS films of this study.[2] Feathers[3] appear in thirty-six films (64%), fur[4] appears in thirty-three films (59%), leather[5] appears in forty-seven films (84%), and shells[6] appear in eight films (14%).

Part III: Disney's Depictions of Clothing and Other Products Made from Animals

From the data presented in Part II, it is clear that products made from animals' bodies are commonplace in WDAS's films. However, most of the time, they are simply background objects, presented without comment. Given that many of these products are not considered controversial in everyday life, it is perhaps unsurprising that WDAS films replicate that attitude. The only clothing product made from animals that has been questioned and criticized by WDAS is fur. However, this has not been the norm throughout Disney's history, as Disney has often used fur clothing to personalize their characters without criticism.

---

[2] Due to the restrictions of animation, it is not possible to accurately record instances of wool and silk in WDAS films. This is because the clothing worn in WDAS films is not usually overly-detailed or explicitly named. Both wool and silk are materials that are difficult to animate using cel-animation, which is how the majority of WDAS films in this study were produced. Therefore, for accuracy, they are not being included here. Furthermore, they are never directly referenced, and the species they are produced from are rarely depicted, so they do not warrant the same level of discussion as other products. Leather is different because WDAS frequently depicts cows (the species leather is produced from) and meat (which cows are often objectified into). Therefore, it is important that leather is included here for consistency.

[3] This specifically means feather products, such as feather quills, feather hats, and so forth. It does not include feathers on living animals.

[4] This specifically means processed fur products, such as a fur coat. It does not include fur on living animals.

[5] This encompasses all depictions that realistically look like leather, such as a leather book strap or leather belt. Of course, it needs to be accepted that given the limits of animation, this may not be entirely accurate.

[6] This refers to processed shells, i.e. without a mollusc, such as Ariel's shell bra.

In the 1950s, Disney produced the live-action television series, *Disneyland*, which was based on the iconic American frontiersman, Davy Crockett. The real Davy Crockett (1786–1836) was a famous hunter and storyteller. For example, in his autobiography, Crockett claimed that he had killed 105 bears in one hunting season (Groneman 2007). In *Disneyland*, Crockett (played by Fess Parker) usually wore his leitmotif, a prominent "coonskin" hat made from real raccoon skin and fur. Given the massive financial success of *Disneyland*, many sequels were made, and each featured Crockett wearing this distinctive fur hat. This led to the hat becoming hugely popular, especially with young boys. During this craze, it was estimated that 5000 of these "coonskin" caps were sold every day (Johnson 2002). However, unlike Fess Parker's, the mass-market version of the hat was made using rabbit or squirrel fur (Mosley 1985: 247–8). This was apparently because the massive demand for the hat outstripped the availability of raccoon fur (Mosley 1985: 247–8). Additionally, to attract the attention of female fans, a "female" version of the hat was also made. This was dubbed the "Polly Crockett" hat (named after Crockett's wife) and was produced using white rabbit fur (Bowers 2014). As mentioned in Part I, fur products are often disliked because of their high cost; however, the Crockett hat was affordable, meaning that it did not evoke wealth resentment in the way that fur products often can. The Davy Crockett craze is notable because this huge use of fur was not commented upon by Disney, even though the scale of animal deaths necessitated for producing these hats seems to be at odds with the anti-fur stance Disney would adopt soon after with *Dalmatians* in 1961. Disney even cashed in on this lucrative trend by depicting Crockett's fur cap on other popular Disney characters, such as Mickey Mouse and Donald Duck (Walker 2015: 24). Traces of Disney's Davy Crockett-craze are still evident today, mainly through their merchandise and at the Disney parks. For example, Disneyland Paris has a Davy Crockett Ranch (*Disneyland Paris* 2019). Disney's Crockett character has not had the longevity of many other Disney characters. To illustrate, in recent years, Disney has re-made several of their most-successful films, such as *The Jungle Book*, *The Lion King*, and so forth. However, at the time of writing, there is no planned remake of Crockett's adventures. Yet Crockett's lack of longevity has not been because he wears fur. In fact, it seems that the "coonskin" cap has remained popular with the public even though the Davy Crockett character has not. For example, the hats are still sold in Disneyland (but they are now entirely faux fur) (Kirk 2013).

WDAS famously adopted an anti-fur stance with 1961's *Dalmatians*, which will be further discussed in Part IV. However, before and after *Dalmatians*, fur was used by Disney and WDAS without criticism, as the Davy Crockett era demonstrates. The WDAS characters that often wear fur clothing are often wealthy female characters, which is reflective of modern fur-wearers. To illustrate, in 1970's *The Aristocats*, Madame Adelaide Bonfamille is lavishly draped in pink fur to establish her wealth, which is later confirmed through the large inheritance she plans to leave her beloved pet cats. In 1977's *The Rescuers,* fur is a symbol of culture and elegance for the film's charming heroine Ms. Bianca, an upper-class diplomat. Another example is 1991's *Beauty and the Beast*, in which a regal fur-trimmed cloak indicates that Belle is an elegant and not impoverished character. Similarly, fur is also worn by WDAS's wealthy male characters to establish their high-status. For example, Prince John in *Robin Hood* (1973) and Jim Dear in *Lady and the Tramp* both wear fur coats, which signifies their wealth. Thus, it is clear that WDAS has often used fur to depict the socio-economic background of their characters.

While most of the fur clothing that has been depicted by WDAS has not been worn by villains, there are a few examples of villainous characters wearing fur in a manner similar to Cruella. For example, Georgette in *Oliver & Company*, The Horned King in *The Black Cauldron*, and Prince John in *Robin Hood* are all villainous characters that wear fur throughout their respective narratives. However, given that WDAS's villains are usually titled or privileged, it makes sense that they are also wealthy (Artz 2004: 130). As highlighted in Part I, many people dislike fur clothing because it is sometimes seen as a vulgar display of wealth (McVeigh 2014). Thus, WDAS perhaps sometimes depicts wealthy villains wearing fur in order to connote that they are anti-social characters.

In contrast, leather appears to be often worn by poorer, more working-class, characters, such as Amos from *The Fox and the Hound* and Robin Hood in *Robin Hood.* For example, Robin Hood appears to wear a leather belt. Additionally, WDAS has often depicted their nomadic and historical characters wearing fur. These depictions also pass no comment on the ethics of using animal's bodies to produce such clothing. For example, in *Hercules* (1997), Hercules is shown wearing the dead carcass of Scar (the antagonistic lion) from *The Lion King* (1994).[7] In another example of nomadic fur wearing, *Brother Bear* (2003) and *Pocahontas* (1995) both depict indigenous people wearing fur and feathers as part of their everyday clothing. They wear these products while living harmoniously around the species that they are produced from. Additionally, it is notable that the animals used for fur in these historical films are "free-range" animals, and not fur-farmed or similar. Similarly, the lost boys in *Peter Pan* wear fur onesies, hats with feathers, and they have fur rugs in their treehouse. In *Peter Pan*, this is to highlight that these characters live nomadic lives away from the city-life that the Darling children came from. The Lost Boys wear and use fur, feathers, and leather, i.e. clothing that they can make themselves using materials from their natural environment. In contrast, the Darling children wear tailored clothing symbolizing the suburban life in London they have left behind. This makes their use of fur justifiable.

As well as using fur to characterize their human and anthropomorphised animal characters, WDAS seems to also use the natural fur on animal characters to make them cuter. For example, Thumper, Flower, and Bambi in *Bambi* all exhibit an exaggerated amount of fur for their species. To illustrate, Flowers' fluffy tail is almost as big as his body. In contrast, villainous animal characters tend to be less fluffy than the species they are based upon. For example, Scar (*The Lion King*) has a greasy and lank mane, which contrasts with the fluffiness of Mufasa and Simba's manes. Thus, it is clear that animals with exaggerated fur tend to be prosocial characters whereas villainous animal characters tend to have less fluffy fur than their species usually has.

To summarize, fur clothing is rarely depicted as a problematic material. Most of WDAS's depictions of fur clothing have not commented on the more controversial side of this product. However, WDAS and Disney films have subtly joked about the fur industry. For example, in *The Fox*

[7] This is an intentional historical reference to the legendary killing of the Nemean lion, which, according to Ancient Greek mythology, was killed by the real Hercules (Stafford 2017: 240). Disney often cameos their animated characters in other films for comedic purposes (*The Telegraph* 2017).

and the Hound (1981), the wearing of fur clothing is directly mocked. Boomer, the comical woodpecker, picks up Tod's bushy fox tail and pretends to wear it as a shawl, similar to how Madame Bonfamille wears fur. A more recent example of Disney joking about the fur industry can be seen in 2012's *Partysaurus Rex*. Earlier, in Pixar's 2001's feature film, *Monsters, Inc.*, the antagonist Randall intimidates the film's protagonist Sully, a furry monster, by telling him that: "Humans skin monsters and make toilet covers out of their fur" (*Monsters, Inc.*, 2001). Eleven years later, a toilet seat made from fur with Sully's distinctive coloration is clearly seen in *Partysaurus Rex*, implying that Sully may have been killed for trivial ends (Lazarus 2015). These jokes demonstrate that while Disney avoids depicting the reality of the fur industry, they are happy to joke about what happens before and after fur production. This is also similar to the points raised in Chap. 1 in regards to farming in *Home on the Range*. These jokes may seem like harmless fun, but they make a mockery of the fur industry. By joking about the production of fur, Disney minimizes the harm that this industry does. It is likely that Disney is doing this because the truth of these industries is far too gruesome to depict accurately, so, as with animal farming, the reality is attenuated in favour of light-hearted jokes.

It is clear that fur has been mostly used by Disney to simply establish character roles or context. As evident from the data in Part II, fur appears in thirty-three of the fifty-six (59%) WDAS films in this study. However, it is most often just background clothing, with no comment or criticism given, just as it was during the "Davy Crockett" craze. Similarly, in the same group of films, leather appears forty-seven times, feathers appear thirty-six times, and shells appear eight times. Yet, unlike fur, the use of these products is always included without passing explicit comment or criticism on the ethics of using animals' bodies to produce those materials. For example, many of the older WDAS films, such as *The Jungle Book* (1967), begin with the opening of a live-action book that appears to be leather-bound. Therefore, WDAS has repeatedly presented leather as a socially-acceptable material to use.

WDAS has used feathers in two main ways: as feather quills and in hats. As with leather, it is often the poorer or working-class characters that seem to have a feather in their cap. Examples of WDAS characters with a single feather in their cap include Robin Hood, Pinocchio, and Peter Pan; none of which are wealthy characters or have high status. For example, Robin Hood lives in a forest and appears to be unemployed. There are a few examples of wealthier characters having a feather in their hat, and in the few instances of this, the feather is usually distinctive, decorated, tailored, and colourful. One example of this is of both Aladdin and Jafar in *Aladdin*. Jafar's feather sits much taller than Pinocchio's and is attached with a jewel. Additionally, the shape of Jafar's feather also suggests that it has been cut or groomed in some way. This could be a metaphor for Jafar's high and privileged status compared to Aladdin.

These points demonstrate that WDAS has criticized animal harm and objectification, but only selectively. WDAS films have not offered explicit critique of the use of leather, feathers, or shells even though they commonly feature in their films. As evidenced in Chap. 1, meat products have often been used by WDAS to characterize toxically-masculine and/or villainous characters. However, it is clear from this chapter that other products made from animals have been presented without criticism most of the time. Similarly, clothing and other products made from animals, have evidently been used throughout WDAS's history to personalize characters, almost-always with little comment on the ethics of the fur industry. These items are usually just character clothing or background objects and are not involved in the main plotline of Disney's stories. Fur clothing has evidently been worn by various types of characters, such as wealthy and nomadic characters. Thus, it is not always associated with villains. For example, Davy Crockett, a pro-social character, almost-always wears a distinctive fur cap. Additionally, Disney has made some subtle jokes about the fur industry that fleetingly acknowledge the brutal reality of the fur industry. These jokes do seem to highlight the morbid fate that animals in the fur industry experience. Disney and WDAS seem to have never passed comment on leather, feathers, and shells even though these products have been widely depicted in more than half of their films.

Part IV: Fur, Leather, and *One Hundred and One Dalmatians*

One Hundred and One Dalmatians (1961) is an example of how to persuasively argue against the fur industry: with humour, extravagance, and no violence towards animals at all. Like PETA's hugely-influential "We'd rather go naked…" anti-fur campaign, *Dalmatians* demonstrates that non-violent portrayals of violent industries can be influential and encourage a practical change in attitudes. *Dalmatians*' success and lasting legacy is mostly thanks to one character: Cruella De Vil. In fact, Cruella is one of the most famous film villains ever, Disney and otherwise (Dockterman and Conniff 2014). However, like other WDAS antagonists adapted from external sources, the nastiness of WDAS's 1961 Cruella pales in comparison to the original Cruella depicted in Dodie Smith's illustrated children's novel *The Hundred and One Dalmatians* (1956). Smith's original text evidently contains much more direct animal harm than Disney's first *Dalmatians* adaptation. It includes stray dogs, abused cats, drowned kittens, and much more serious danger for the hunted Dalmatian puppies. For example, when discussing her unloved Persian cat, Smith's Cruella proudly boasts:

> I've drowned dozens and dozens of my cat's kittens. She always chooses some wretched alley-cat for their father. So they're never worth keeping. (Cruella in Smith's text (Smith 2010: 14))

Much of this direct animal harm was adapted out, attenuated, or handled with humour by WDAS, which chose to only ever imply harm.

Cruella's appearance was dramatically different in Smith's text too. In Smith's text (which was illustrated), Cruella was noticeably prettier, younger, and more elegant than she would later be in the WDAS adaptation. WDAS's iconic 1961 Cruella character was designed by one of Disney's "nine old men", Marc Davis. Davis also animated the ugly sisters in *Cinderella* (1950) and Maleficent from *Sleeping Beauty* (1959), so he had a strong history of creating memorable female villains (Gartler 2015). Davis evidently experimented with Cruella's look. In some early sketches, she was much prettier and younger than she would later be. As was common with WDAS at the time, live actors performed the film's storyboard to inspire the realistic appearance and movements of the animated characters (Thomas and Johnston 1981). It was after this live-storyboarding that Davis created the final iconic look of WDAS's famous Cruella character. WDAS's Cruella is skeletal with unnatural, zombie-like, grey skin. She is often smoking a long thin cigarette. Audiences instinctively prefer characters that are circular in design, such as Mickey Mouse (Artz 2004: 118). This is why animated villains are usually skinny and tall, as is the case with Cruella. This design of villainous character can also be seen with the evil queen (*Snow White*), Lady Tremaine (*Cinderella*), and Maleficent (*Sleeping Beauty*). Additionally, by making Cruella older, she is not neotenous, which also makes her instinctively less likeable. Young, or young-looking, characters are favoured over older characters (Gould 1977). This is why WDAS's villains are usually the oldest characters in their narratives. Thus, Cruella's appearance alone makes her instinctively unlikeable, which makes her appear villainous before she has even expressed her desire to harm puppies.

Cruella is infamous for her selfishness, dramatics, and greed. This is what makes her character, and thus the film, so comical. As highlighted in the previous chapter, there are two types of villains: the repellent and the intriguing (Forbes 2011: 13–27). Like a pantomime dame,[8] Cruella is an intriguing villain because she is comical, but also because her villainous aims are unsuccessful. This is similar to many of WDAS's other intriguing villains, such as Captain Hook (*Peter Pan*) and Ursula (*The Little Mermaid*). The attempted harms of these villains are also unsuccessful, which is what makes them intriguing rather than repellent. While Cruella is less cruel in WDAS's adaptation than in Smith's original, she is still the text's main villain, and she still repeatedly expresses a desire to harm animals for her own selfish needs. When Cruella is first introduced, she carelessly drives through a flock of peaceful white birds (which are unharmed by the incident). Then, after seeing the new-born Dalmatian

[8] British pantomime is a typical a family theatre show with comedy and music. Such shows usually feature a "pantomime dame", a matronly, camp, older women that is played by a male. Further information can be found in: Sladen 2015: 80–89.

puppies, she is disgusted by their spot-less appearance. She labels them as "mongrels" and "horrid little white rats" upon seeing that they do not yet have their signature black Dalmatian spots. After Roger refuses to sell the puppies to Cruella, she angrily exclaims "Do as you like with them, drown them!" She then aggressively leaves, screaming and smashing a window pane as she loudly exits. Despite this aggression, and her gruesome plans, Cruella seems unwilling to directly harm the puppies herself. However, she is happy to suggest violent ways for others to do it. For example, she instructs her hired helpers (Jasper and Horace) to "Poison them, drown them, bash them in the head! You got any chloroform?" Yet despite not being directly violent towards any animals, Cruella is violent towards the human characters. For example, she slaps Jasper and Horace after seeing that they have not yet killed the puppies, which is more violent than she ever is towards the puppies. Thus, even though *Dalmatians* is a film about direct animal harm, no direct animal harm is ever presented in the film. The most harm the dogs experience is during their difficult journey in the snow storm, which is no direct fault of Cruella's. In fact, most of the on-screen violence and peril affects the would-be animal harmers (Cruella, Jasper, and Horace), rather than the animals. The dogs do face neglect and peril, such as being carelessly put into a bag, but never violence. Furthermore, the small amount of mistreatment the puppies experience is kept off-screen and temporary, as is often the case in WDAS films.

Cruella De Vil is probably one of the Anglo-American world's most famous would-be direct animal harmers despite the fact that she never actually harms any animals. However, while some of Cruella's character traits, such as her lack of empathy and choice of target animal are also frequently evident in real direct animal abusers, most of her character does not fit the profile of a person who directly harms animals (Marino and Mountain 2015: 5–21; Flynn 2012: 23). Research into people who directly harm animals has claimed that direct animal harm is overwhelmingly committed by individual teenage males from lower socio-economic backgrounds, usually as a result of mental instability (Flynn 2012: 10–30). Therefore, Cruella, as a mature wealthy female, does not fit the typical demographic of a direct animal harmer. However, she does perfectly characterize people that harm animals *indirectly*, i.e. people who buy fur products. As highlighted in Part I of this chapter, in the Anglo-American context, fur is a product that is mainly aimed at wealthy Anglo-American women. This is one of the reasons why it is so disliked compared to similar products made from animals' bodies.

The other characters who attempt to harm animals in *Dalmatians* are Cruella's hapless dog thieves, Jasper and Horace. Like Cruella, these two inject amusement into the story with their comic incompetence and slapstick humour. Unlike Cruella, they are working-class men. This is conveyed through their cockney-rhyming slang, inexpensive clothing, and motivation (they are only helping Cruella for money). This stops them from being repellent villains. Thus, without Cruella, Jasper and Horace would likely not attempt to harm animals directly. Also like Cruella, these two are only ever violent towards humans, despite their attempts to harm animals. For example, when kidnapping the puppies, Jasper and Horace are very aggressive towards the housekeeper, Nanny. They violently overpower her and lock her in the attic in order to steal the puppies. This is the most purposefully violent these two are in the whole narrative, and it is towards a human character, not an animal. After overpowering Nanny, Horace and Jasper put the puppies in a bag off-screen, showing a clear lack of concern for the dogs' welfare. However, the thieves later keep the stolen puppies in an old mansion, which does not accurately reflect the harsh conditions on real fur farms. While in the mansion, the puppies are seen enjoying several luxuries, such as television and snacks. Thus, they are not caged, neglected, or mistreated by Jasper and Horace. Furthermore, Jasper and Horace are reluctant to harm the puppies and only attempt to do so after Cruella aggressively insists. Jasper then says: "I'll pop 'em on the head, you do the skinning" before arguing with Horace about who will do the puppy-skinning. While this dispute occurs, the puppies safely escape from the mansion unharmed. As Jasper and Horace chase the dogs, the dogs repeatedly overpower them in a slapstick fashion. For example, Jasper and Horace are bit on the bottom, fall into a fire, are thrown against a barn wall, and, eventually, the mansion roof falls in on them. They survive the violence, but they do not recapture the dogs, all of which escape safely.

It is also worth noting that even though Cruella is pro-fur, the other human and animal characters are not anti-fur. At the beginning of the film, Pongo (the Dalmatian) is searching for a girlfriend for his owner Roger. As he searches for a suitable partner, he sees several women walking their dogs. Most of these women are wearing fur. For example, the poodle-owner appears to be wearing poodle fur, and so forth. This is a comical scene that suggests that dog-owners look like their dogs. The ethics of the fur industry are not alluded to at all during this scene. This is significant because the production of fur is later what Pongo and his Dalmatian family almost become victims of. Additionally, upon hearing Cruella talk about fur, Anita (the owner of the Dalmatians) claims that "I'd like a nice fur, but there are so many other things…" This implies that Anita is not against the idea of wearing fur, she merely believes that there are better ways to spend money. Additionally, Nanny, the sweet-natured housekeeper, appears to have a leather handbag. In fact, there are numerous objects that appear to be leather throughout the film, and they are presented without comment. For example, in one scene, the puppies are sat on what appears to be a leather sofa, highlighting the stark difference in attitudes towards fur and leather products. This ultimately highlights the problem with *Dalmatians*: its replication of speciesist attitudes. The intentions of the story – i.e. to highlight the cruelty of wearing fur – are laudable. However, the problem is that this film reflects, and thus normalizes, speciesist attitudes. *Dalmatians* suggests that it is permissible to objectify some species, such as cattle, but not others, such as anthropomorphised, individualized, neotenized dogs. As highlighted in Part I, the fur trade is one of the most-criticized areas of global animal objectification even though it has far fewer victims than other industries that harm animals, such as the meat and dairy industry. If *Dalmatians* was about Cruella chasing cows to make a leather coat, it is unlikely it would have conveyed such an influential message. This is similar to the logical inconsistencies towards hunting and fishing within *Brother Bear*, as highlighted in the previous chapter.

After the release of *Dalmatians* in 1961, real fur became noticeably less fashionable in the Anglo-American world (North 2000: 17–8). Additionally, supporters of fur directly criticized the film. For example, the now-defunct pro-fur publication *Fur Age Weekly* claimed that *Dalmatians* offered children "a gruesome picture" of the fur industry (Urquhart 1991). The anti-fur trend exploded in the 1980s alongside the birth of PETA, which focused many of their eye-catching campaigns on the cruelty of fur production, such as their 1994 "We'd rather go naked…" campaign (McVeigh 2014). *Dalmatians*' anti-fur message is still used today in animal welfare campaigns. For example, "Furry Tales" (2014) is a set of 2014 graphic designs that depicts various popular Disney characters, such as the Dalmatian puppies and Bambi, as skinned, bleeding, and in distress, in order to highlight the suffering usually involved in fur production (Dearden 2014). However, while sales of fur declined after the release of *Dalmatians*, Cruella's popularity did not. WDAS's ugly, inelegant, dramatic Cruella proved to be much more popular than Smith's original. In 1967, Smith released a sequel novel, *The Starlight Barking*, in which Cruella appears only briefly (Smith 1967). The text follows where the previous novel finished, yet during Cruella's fleeting appearance, she is asleep. However, as was clear from the 1961 WDAS film, Cruella was the star of this story, and unsurprisingly, Disney has yet to show any interest in adapting Smith's sequel. Yet Disney has since adapted Smith's original text again, and they have also written their own sequels to this story. These adaptations and appropriations have each centred around WDAS's 1961 Cruella character, rather than Smith's crueller and younger version. This demonstrates that despite Cruella's villainy, she is the story's most memorable character. In 1996, Cruella's character was brought to life in the live-action *Dalmatians* remake (*The Numbers* 2019a). As with the 1961 adaptation, Cruella's puppy kill count remained at zero. The critical and financial success of the 1996 remake encouraged Disney and other media companies to produce more adaptations and appropriations of this story, all of which have focused upon WDAS's Cruella rather than the dogs or Smith's Cruella. In 1997, Disney Television produced the animated show, *101 Dalmatians: The Series* (*IMDB* 2019). Three years later, in 2003, another animated sequel, *101 Dalmatians II: Patch's London Adventure* was released by Disneytoon Studios. Cruella was once-again the main villain in this text. In 2009, the story was adapted into a stage musical: *The 101 Dalmatians Musical* (not by Disney). The theatrical role of Cruella was played by Rachel York, who, like Glenn Close before her, quickly established herself as a "huge animal lover" while promoting the show (Scherer 2009). More recently, Cruella also came to life in the Disney Channel's *Descendants* movie (2015) (Snetiker 2014). *Descendants* features Cruella as a stand-alone character in an entirely new story, which again highlights her memorability compared to the original story's other characters. Unsurprisingly, Cruella's adaptation journey is not over yet. Disney is currently developing yet another Cruella-focused live-action film, aptly titled *Cruella*, which is due for release in 2021 (*IMDB* 2018b). Further to the media mentioned above, Cruella has inspired books, video games, songs, merchandise, and more (for example: *Shop Disney* 2019c). Therefore, Cruella is undoubtedly one of WDAS's most revived fictional villains, despite her socially-unacceptable attitude towards the welfare of dogs. Of course, there are many other notable villains that have also been revived several times, such as The Joker, The Terminator, and Freddy Krueger. However, Cruella seems to be one of the very few female villains that has been repeatedly revived in such a way.

There are three patterns are evident with the post-1961 Cruella characters. First, they are all based upon WDAS's much-less violent 1961 Cruella, rather than Dodie Smith's Cruella. This is true even in non-Disney productions, such as the 2009 stage musical. Second, Cruella never actually kills *any* puppies in any of these adaptations. Her on-screen puppy kill count remains at zero, despite the many chances she has had to kill animals, and the many times she has threatened to. Third, all of Cruella's live-action actors have been very vocal about their *off-screen* love of animals, particularly dogs, which seems incongruous with Cruella's personality, yet essential for media promotion (Stanton 2017). It seems clear that Cruella's attempted animal harm has to be thwarted for the character to be funny, which may also help explain why Dodie Smith's much crueller Cruella has been eschewed in favour of Disney's. However, this unique clause seems exclusive to the Cruella character. For example, actors that play serial killers are not expected to confirm that they are not *really* serial killers. As will be demonstrated in Chap. 5, audiences tend to be sensitive towards violence involving animals in film. Documented instances of animal harm can destroy a film's reputation, which is why films are expected to say that "No animals were harmed…" during their credits. This is perhaps why actors playing Cruella are expected to confirm that Cruella's character is fake. Looking at all of Cruella's media appearances, it certainly seems unusual that despite her violent intentions and reputation, she does not actually ever harm any animals, on or off-screen. However, this is what makes her character engaging, rather than repellent.

Cruella does not murder any animals across her many Disney adaptations, even though she has had many chances to do so. In contrast, so many animals are killed during the production of fur clothing that the numbers cannot be accurately recorded. The fur industry is real; it is not fictional, animated, or exaggerated. In fact, its existence is minimized and ridiculed by mainstream cultural representations, such as *Dalmatians*. Furthermore, real fur wearers are normal, everyday people. Additionally, they rarely have to hunt the animals they are wearing because most fur clothing comes ready-made from fur farms, which are notorious for their inattention to animal welfare (Meredith 2013). Moreover, the species used by the fur industry are also misrepresented in this text. *Dalmatians* suggests that animals hunted for fur are free-range baby pet animals, which is not typically the case. As highlighted in Part I, the majority of fur comes from rodents on fur farms (*Fur Free Alliance* 2018). The reality of the fur industry has never been depicted by Disney, despite their numerous adaptations of this fur-centred story. If anything, *Dalmatians* (1961) and its many adaptations could be seen as a compliment to the fur industry because it places the blame onto unrealistic fictional characters, such as Cruella. This can also be compared to the ways in which WDAS has attenuated and minimized the reality of animal farming, as was demonstrated in Chap. 1.

However, WDAS's wholesome, funny animation, and its many adaptations, have been effective and lucrative precisely *because* they do not depict violence towards animals, only the threat of it. If *Dalmatians* had contained violence towards puppies, it likely would have had a different legacy, as is indicated by other films that have contained depictions of violence against animals. As highlighted in Part I of this chapter and elsewhere in this book, PETA's shocking exposé films often receive negative reactions from both critics and viewers (Burt 2002: 171). In fact, it is usually argued that the grisly violence of PETA's campaigns makes these campaigns less-engaging, which undermines their aims.[9] In contrast, *Dalmatians* (1961) and its many adaptations are entertaining films with

---

[9] A brief overview of some of PETA's controversial campaigns can be found in: Yount 2008: 15–17.

happy and optimistic endings.[10] This happiness and optimism provides hope, which is what makes *Dalmatians* so engaging.

Walt apparently disliked *Dalmatians* because of its poor-quality animation in comparison to WDAS's earlier films (Pallant 2011: 70). Despite this, *Dalmatians* has become one of Disney's most revered stories. Counterintuitively, Cruella herself is today one of Disney's most famous characters despite her sinister intentions. This is because she never actually kills or harms animals, she only ever threatens to. Cruella, as a character, is engaging and thus intriguing because she is comical and unrealistic. *Dalmatians* could reasonably be considered the most recognizable anti-fur films ever, but its depiction of the fur industry and other products made from animals is problematic. Because of this, *Dalmatians* ultimately serves as a compliment to the fur industry because it is the Anglo-American world's most famous anti-fur film, yet it minimizes the harsh reality of the fur industry. Additionally, it leaves other products derived from animals, such as leather and dairy products, unquestioned and thus they are depicted as socially-acceptable.

Conclusion

The evidence presented throughout this chapter suggests that Karl Lagerfeld is right: the discussion of fur is childish. It is childish because it lacks critical thinking and is underpinned by illogical speciesist biases, as Part I demonstrated. Disney, like the public, is speciesist and inconsistent with their concern towards animals. The Davy Crockett era implies that Disney was happy to sell massive amounts of fur. In contrast, *Dalmatians* and its many adaptations imply that puppies should be protected from the fur industry, but this film does not extend this protection onto other species, such as cows and birds. Products made from animals' bodies are usually just background objects without criticisms or compliments in Disney media. Therefore, it could not be said that *Dalmatians* is a brave

[10] The 1961 *Dalmatians* film did, however, receive criticism and complaints for a scene in which the Dalmatian puppies nurse from some happy free-range dairy cows. This scene was cut from the film's theatrical release in many countries as the sight of animated cow teats was deemed offensive (Cochrane 2014).

or ambitious text; it is simply another example of Disney following consumer trends to their advantage.

Disney's upcoming *Dalmatians* adaptation (due 2021) focusses on a younger Cruella. As is clear from PETA's "We'd rather go naked…" campaign and the success of Disney's various Cruella characters, using sexy, dramatic, and funny characters has the potential to shape public opinions. Therefore, if this new adaptation still has the original text's anti-fur message, it may continue to discourage people from wearing fur. However, that is likely to be as far as the film's pro-animal message will go. It is unlikely to challenge the issues that affect a far greater number of animals, such as the meat and leather industries. As demonstrated here, Disney clearly has limits to their concern for animal welfare that are in line with the public's social-acceptance of the issue.

This chapter has focused mostly on fur products as that is where the previous foci of this discussion has been. However, given that the production of fur is now mostly socially-unacceptable (and even in some countries illegal) in the Anglo-American context, it is perhaps time for animal rights' campaigns to begin opposing leather and other products made from animals, as the production of these products affects a far greater number of animals. Up to now, campaigns against the production of leather have been ineffective, but this is perhaps because of the off-putting violence and hopelessness that they exhibit. As this chapter has demonstrated, the most influential anti-fur campaigns have been non-violent and optimistic, so this is how anti-leather campaigns should undoubtedly proceed in order to be more successful with their aims.

4

Pets and Working Animals in WDAS Films

Peter Singer famously differentiated between "the human" and "the person" by arguing that some non-human animals can be individual persons, and that not all humans are necessarily persons. Singer believes that for an animal to be a person, it must possess memories, a family, and unique behaviours (1995: 180–183, 197–198). He argues that some humans, such as babies and the severely mentally-disabled, cannot be persons because they are unable to meaningfully possess these individual qualities. Thus, according to Singer's reasoning, some pet animals can be more of a person than a human can. Yet some other animals, such as working animals, are excluded from the category of "persons" because they are forced into monotonous, isolated, working routines which mean that they have little chance to develop familial bonds. Therefore, while animals have the capacity for personhood, their ability to develop that capacity is limited by human intervention.

To explore these ideas further, this chapter will examine depictions of pets and working animals in WDAS films. These two types of characters are widespread in WDAS films; their prevalence is perhaps reflective of reality since these animals have been so common in everyday human life and history. Part I will explore the history of and common ethical

R. R. Stanton, *The Disneyfication of Animals*, The Palgrave Macmillan Animal Ethics Series, https://doi.org/10.1007/978-3-030-49316-5_4

objections towards pets and working animals. Part II will document how often pet-keeping and using animals for labour have been depicted in WDAS films. Then, Part III will examine and highlight any patterns evident in the data, along with the types of direct and indirect harm that these characters face in WDAS films. Finally, Part IV will analyse *Lady and the Tramp* (1955), a WDAS film that focusses on pet animals but also features working animals. This chapter will conclude by claiming that direct harm towards non-villainous pets appears to be acknowledged more than any other type of animal harm in WDAS films. In contrast, working animals tend to face routine physical harm as part of their role, yet such harms are rarely criticized or even acknowledged. This chapter will conclude by arguing that this disparity in concern towards the welfare of working animals and pets is the result of speciesist biases.

Part I: The History and Ethics of Pets and Working Animals

Throughout this chapter, the term "working animal" will refer to an animal that has been domesticated or trained to perform physical labour—transporting humans, carrying loads, providing protection, and so forth—for human benefit.[1] As Part II will demonstrate, working animals have been depicted in 54% of WDAS films. However, given their importance and prevalence within human history, this is perhaps not surprising. It is believed that humans have used animals for labour since before the advent of agriculture. For example, when humans were hunter-gatherers, they trained dogs to assist with hunting (Sullivan 2012: 54). Today, it is believed that cattle are the most common species of working animal globally, followed by horses, donkeys, and then mules (Starkey 2000: 478). It is notable that working animals are more commonly male

[1] The term "working animal" can sometimes include animals that are kept only to produce food and/ or clothing, such as cows. However, since farm animals were discussed in Chap. 1, they will not be discussed again here. Similarly, animals that provide entertainment for humans, such as circus animals, will be discussed in Chap. 5, so they will not be discussed in this chapter.

since they are often stronger than females, but also because they cannot produce dairy, so they are often surplus on farms (Starkey 2000: 478).[2]

There are four common criticisms of making animals work. First, they are unwaged (Hribal 2003: 436). Second, working animals have physically-challenging lives (*SPANA* 2019b). Third, once they are too old to work, they are often killed unceremoniously (Barnett 2006). Fourth, working animals are unable to consent to the roles assigned to them. Therefore, working animals experience similar welfare issues to farmed animals. Yet despite experiencing routine harms, there have been few campaigns focussed on improving the welfare of working animals. This may be because working animals, such as donkeys, do not tend to score on the higher-level of the socio-zoological scale, meaning that their welfare is instinctively less concerning to humans. This lack of concern may also be because working animals are not often individualized. Animals used for labour usually work in large groups of their species, which elicits the "collapse of compassion" response. To illustrate, in WDAS films, horses usually exist in the background of the story in large, non-anthropomorphised, groups. This can be seen in *Sleeping Beauty*, *The Little Mermaid*, and *The Princess and the Frog*, amongst many other examples. Furthermore, only a small amount of cultural representations have accurately depicted the harsh lives that working animals experience. For example, Anna Sewell's 1877 novel *Black Beauty* questioned the ethics of forcing horses to perform hard labour for long periods of time. This text is directly credited with the widespread removal of a leather-strap that held working horses' heads unnaturally high (Dorré 2002: 157–78). This suggests that if cultural representations did challenge the harms entailed in making animals work, there could be more consideration towards these animals. This highlights why WDAS's depictions of working animals are important and warrant study. The exception to this lack of concern for working animals is dogs. Although dogs are sometimes given jobs, they are still usually individualized, and their treatment outside of labour is often much more considerate than the care provided to

[2] This chapter will not explore the history of working animals in-depth as the focus of this text is WDAS films. A more-detailed overview on the history of working animals can be found at: https://spana.org/thenandnow/ (accessed: 4 April 2019). SPANA (The Society for the Protection of Animals Abroad) is a British charity that focuses on the welfare of working animals.

donkeys, for example. To illustrate, there are several charities specifically for the welfare of guide dogs, such as the Guide Dogs Association (*Guide Dogs* 2019) and Assistance Dogs UK (*Assistance Dogs* 2019). Additionally, dogs do not tend to perform physically challenging labour, such as transporting goods, with rare exceptions such as snow dogs. However, if dogs had not originally been used as working animals, it is unlikely that they would have developed strong relations with humans and become the most popular species of pet, which they are believed to be today (Borgi and Cirulli 2015, 2016).

As noted above, humans have lived alongside animals for thousands of years. However, these animals were kept to provide labour, not companionship (McRobbie 2017). Animals that lived alongside humans in the past were not viewed as affectionately as they are today. For example, in the Middle Ages, dogs that died were often eaten rather than buried (McRobbie 2017). Pet-keeping, as it is known today, is a recent phenomenon that appears to have arisen alongside disposable incomes (McRobbie 2017). Today, pets[3] are highly valued animals when compared to many other categories of animal, such as working animals and farmed animals. For example, 90% of British people claim that pets are a part of their family (McRobbie 2017). There are three reasons for this: pets are usually higher-order species, they are visible in everyday human life, and they are individualized. It is estimated that 46% of UK households and 62% of US households have pets (Shuttlewood et al. 2016: 181). Therefore, pet-keeping is today very common in Anglo-American culture, and, as Part II will demonstrate, it is a commonly-depicted practice within WDAS films.

In quantitative terms, fish are the most common pet (Brown 2015: 1). However, several studies have found that both adults and children listed dogs are their favourite species of pet (Borgi and Cirulli 2015, 2016). Singer argues that humans express concern for dogs because that is the species that humans have the most direct experience with (2009: 30). It is commonly believed that dogs were the first animal domesticated by humans. This was to help humans with practical tasks, such as hunting (Sullivan 2012: 54). Yet today, the majority of modern dog-owners own

[3] Within this chapter and wider book, "pet" will refer to a non-human animal that lives with a human in the human's home or garden.

a dog for companionship rather than for practical reasons (Zawistowski and Reid 2016: 228). Dogs are still used by humans as guide dogs, police dogs, guard dogs, and so forth. Yet unlike other animals that work, such as horses, dogs usually live with humans when not working and after retirement (for example: *Retired Police Canine Foundation* 2019). There are many Disney films based on true, or plausible, stories of the love and loyalty dogs exhibit towards humans, such as *Homeward Bound* (1963, 1993), *Old Yeller* (1957), *Lady and the Tramp* (1955), and *Bolt* (2008). As Part II will highlight, dogs are widespread characters in WDAS films, especially as pets. Across the fifty-six films in this study, dogs are depicted in thirty-three films, which is more often than any other species. Furthermore, some of the official Disney hotels even allow pet dogs (not just service dogs) to stay with their human owners (*Disney World* 2019). This privilege is currently offered to no other species. However, despite their domestication, dogs still exhibit behaviour that humans consider disgusting (Serpell 2016: 310). For example, their olfactory preoccupations, uninhibited sexually promiscuous behaviour, and fondness for human garbage are often considered embarrassing to humans (Serpell 2016: 310). This is likely why these traits are rarely depicted when dogs are anthropomorphised. Additionally, these behaviours are discouraged in pet and working dogs (Serpell 2016: 310). It is mostly the supposedly human-like behaviours of dogs (such as loyalty) that have been amplified and celebrated. Thus, while dogs are well-liked by humans, their likeability depends on their behaviour.

Even though pets seem to be treated better than many other animals, such as working animals, there are several objections to pet-keeping. Some of the most common criticisms are aimed towards pet shops, puppy farms, and forced inbreeding (McRobbie 2017).[4] Certain practices, such as declawing, have even inspired their own campaigns and as a result have been banned in some countries. For example, declawing is banned in Germany (*PETA* 2019k). There are also several objections to pet-keeping from a more philosophical angle. For example, animals become pets because the human wants them, and not vice-versa (McRobbie 2017).

[4] This chapter will not discuss these issues in great detail. Further information on the ethics of pet-keeping can be found in: *Run, Spot, Run: The Ethics of Keeping Pets* by Jessica Pierce (2016).

Therefore, pet ownership is seen as anthropocentric because it is based entirely on the human's desires and choices. Furthermore, it is claimed that pet owners often have insufficient knowledge about the natural environment and behaviour of the species they own (Endenburg and Vorstenbosch 1992: 129). These objections suggest that there has been much more critical thinking in this area than many other areas of animal welfare. These points also imply that there is more appreciation of the sentience of pets compared to other animals. Because the ethics of pet ownership have elicited greater concern than the ethics of working animals, people who display concern for the welfare of pets are sometimes labelled speciesist (Spencer et al. 2006: 17–25). This is because criticisms of pet-keeping, such as those highlighted above, are rarely allayed at practices involving lower-order animals, such as working animals. For example, while puppy farms are heavily criticized (for example: *The Kennel Club* 2019b), the farming of most other animals receives very little attention, as was highlighted in Chap. 1.

It has been repeatedly found that depictions of animals in film strongly influence the species and breeds that people subsequently choose as pets. This has been dubbed the "Disney effect" by newspapers and researchers. Despite its name, the "Disney effect" is evidenced to occur with other film companies too. For example, sales of Collies significantly rose after the release of Metro-Goldwyn-Mayer's *Lassie Come Home* in 1943 (Ghirlanda et al. 2014). The "Disney effect" is evidenced to occur with both live-action and animated films (Garner 1996). For example, after Disney's live-action *The Shaggy Dog* (1959), sales of Old English Sheepdogs rose by 100% (Carter 2014). After 1961's *Dalmatians*, demand for Dalmatians doubled even though the film was animated (Garner 1996). However, this surge in Dalmatian adoptions became a problem because, despite their leisurely behaviour in the 1961 WDAS film, Dalmatians are high-energy dogs. The demanding nature of Dalmatians resulted in many pet-owners giving their new dogs to shelters (Jeppley 2010). Therefore, many dogs were abandoned because they did not live up to their anthropomorphised depiction in WDAS's *Dalmatians*. This also affected Dalmatians in the long-term as this surge in demand led to over-breeding and irresponsible breeding. This reduced the overall quality of the breed and was claimed to have resulted in genetic problems for the dogs (Jeppley 2010). The "Disney Effect" is believed to last for around a decade after a film's release; if this is correct, it has the potential to affect a significant number of real animals (Carter 2014). Because of the "Disney effect", animal welfare organizations have become pro-active with the release of subsequent animal-centred films. For example, before the release of Disney's live-action *Dalmatians* remake in 1996, several organizations urged the public not to buy Dalmatians impulsively (Garner 1996). For example, The British Dalmatian Club urged their members to distribute flyers that said: "Seen the film? Read the book? Want the dog? Wait" (Garner 1996). Disney was evidently aware of the "Disney effect" as *Dalmatians* (1996) encouraged their viewers to adopt dogs responsibly during the film's credits (Sheen 2005: 237). Yet despite this acknowledgement, Disney released *Dalmatians* at Christmas, which generated further criticism (Garner 1996). This is because it is well known that dogs are often bought impulsively at Christmas (*Dogs Trust* 2018). The "Disney effect" is evidenced to affect other species too, not just dogs. For example, after the release of Disney-Pixar's *Finding Nemo* (2003), sales of clown fish soared (Jeppley 2010). As with dogs, this was problematic from a welfare perspective as clown fish are much more demanding than traditional pet fish (Jeppley 2010). However, it has also been argued that the "Disney effect" can benefit real animals. For example, it has been argued that Disney-Pixar's *Ratatouille* (2007) changed viewpoints on rats for the better (Jeppley 2010). The "Disney effect" further demonstrates why WDAS's depictions animals, particularly pet animals, are important and warrant study: because WDAS's portrayals of animals have the potential to affect huge numbers of the real species that they are based upon.

Further to the Disney effect, it has been proven that children are influenced by depictions of animals in cultural representations. For example, Kidd and Kidd (1990) found that what children learned about animals from the media heavily affected their subsequent attitudes and behaviours towards their own pets. Similarly, Valkenburg (2004) suggests that the way children treat animals in reality is influenced by cultural representations (2004: 25). Additionally, Anderson and Henderson's 2005 study claimed that depictions of animals in the media can influence children for life (2005: 301). These studies demonstrate that care is needed when depicting animals, especially in media viewed by children. It would be fair to suggest that the children who participated in those studies had been in direct contact with every species they liked or disliked; thus, it is reasonable to conclude that some of the speciesist prejudices they held had developed from their engagement with cultural representations. Therefore, the attitudes reflected in cultural representations, such as WDAS films, are important because they are evidenced to influence how children view and treat animals in reality (Kidd and Kidd 1990; Valkenburg 2004; Anderson and Henderson 2005).

To conclude Part I, it is clear that pet-keeping and using animals for labour are two practices that have been a significant part of human history and culture. However, the animals involved in these two practices face different forms of discrimination and harm. For example, a significant number of working animals have physically-challenging lives and are not treated as individuals, which prohibits them from being considered "persons". In contrast, pets are usually individualized and are offered a high-level of respect. Some animals, such as dogs and cats, have shifted from being predominantly working animals to pets. This is "progress" because pets commonly experience less harm than working animals. Pets are commonly given "personhood", which working animals are not. Other species, such as horses, have remained as working animals and are rarely considered to be pets. It is generally socially-unacceptable to harm pets; this is evident from the many campaigns and laws that exist to protect them (for example: *PETA* 2019e). In contrast, there are few laws and campaigns for the welfare of working animals. Moreover, very few cultural representations have explored, questioned, or even individualized, the lives of working animals. In contrast, pets are commonly depicted favourably in cultural representations, wherein they are commonly anthropomorphised and individualized. However, this has led to the "Disney effect". The "Disney effect" refers to Disney's influence on the pets subsequently sold, and, as a result, sometimes abandoned, in reality. The remainder of this chapter will now examine how pets and working animals have been depicted in WDAS films.

Part II: Data

A full list of all depictions of pets and working animals in WDAS films (1937–2016) can be found on pages 131–139 of the appendixes.

Combined Numbers

- Animal shelters/pounds are featured in three films (5%).
- Pet shops are featured in three films (5%).
- Pets are featured in thirty-two films (57%). Across these thirty-two films, there are fifty-four different pets or same-species groups of pets.
- Working animals are featured in thirty films (54%). Across these thirty films, there are forty different working animal characters or same-species groups of characters.

WDAS's Pets

- Fifteen films feature cats as pets (27%). Fifteen films feature dogs as pets (27%). Four films feature goldfish as pets (7%). Two films feature lizards and ravens as pets (4%). Angel fish, chickens, crocodiles, crickets, falcons, foxes, goats, hamsters, hummingbirds, monkeys, owls, parrots, pigs, raccoons, snakes, and tigers are each depicted in one film as a pet (2% each).
- Pets are mammals in thirty-seven films (69%). Birds are pets in seven films (13%). Fish are pets in five films (9%). Reptiles are pets in four films (7%). Insects are pets once (2%).
- In thirty-six cases (67%), pets are anthropomorphised but mute. In thirteen cases, pets are heavily-anthropomorphised (24%). In five instances, pets are not anthropomorphised at all (9%).
- Twenty-nine pets are male (54%), eight are female (15%), thirteen are without a clear gender (24%), and four exist in mixed-gender groups of their species (7%).
- Forty-one pets have names (76%), and thirteen are nameless (24%).
- Nine of WDAS's pets are villainous (17%).

Working Animals

- Twenty-six films feature horses as working animals (65%). Five films feature dogs as working animals (12.5%). Two films feature donkeys, cattle, and/or llamas (5%). Camels, deer, and reindeer appear in one film each (2.5% each). Therefore, all of WDAS's working animals are mammals.
- In eleven films, working animals are anthropomorphised, but mute (27.5%). In twenty-five films, working animals are not anthropomorphised at all (62.5%). In four films, working animals are heavily anthropomorphised and can speak (10%).
- In thirty-six films, working animals are genderless (90%). In three films, they are male (7.5%). In one film, they are female (2.5%).
- The purposes of working animals are as follows: animals are used for riding/human transport in twenty-nine films (72.5%); animals are used for carrying goods in six films (15%); animals are used for animal hunting or as a police animal in two films each (5%); animals are used for protection in one film (2.5%).
- In thirty-six cases (90%), working animals are nameless. In four cases (10%), most of the working-animals have names.

Part III: WDAS's Pets and Working Animals

As the other chapters of this book have demonstrated, Walt had a fondness for animals that helped shaped the unique, animal-centred, output of the Disney studios (Wills 2017: 26). As detailed in Chap. 1, Walt spent his early life on a farm populated with a small number of animals that he individualized and anthropomorphised. Both Walt and Roy found it difficult to leave their beloved farm because of the animals they had to leave behind. Roy remembered one animal in particular:

> We had a little six-month colt [that] was sold and tied up to a buggy and taken away, and Walt and I both cried. Later on that day… we were down in town and here was this farmer and his rig hitched up to the hitching rack and our little colt tied on behind… and the damn little colt saw us when we were across the street and he whinnied and whinnied and reared back on his tie-down, and we went over and hugged him and cried over him… That was the last we saw of him. [sic] (Roy, in: Barrier 2007: 17)

Anecdotes such as this one perhaps help to explain why animal characters were such a significant part of Walt's later work. It also suggests that Walt felt sympathy with unconventional species of animals, such as colts, which are not often individualized because they are usually considered working animals. This suggests that Walt perhaps viewed working animals more affectionately than most people, at least when he was a child. It is also well-documented that Walt was fond of mice and would keep them as pets:

> I used to find them [mice] in my waste basket in the mornings. I kept several in a cage on my drawing board and enjoyed watching their antics. (Walt, in: Barrier 2007: 56)

This quote demonstrates that Walt enjoyed keeping mice as pets, but also that he did not question the ethics of keeping "pet" animals caged. Walt seemed to have placed his enjoyment of "watching their antics" above the freedom of the mice. As Part I highlighted, selfishness is a common criticism of pet-keeping. This again demonstrates that while Walt liked animals, many of his actions were shaped by anthropocentric views. These anthropocentric ideas are reflected in WDAS films, which celebrate certain species of animals, but only those that dote on humans (such as dogs) or act human (i.e. are heavily-anthropomorphised).

It is clear that WDAS has depicted working animals and pets in very different ways, so this chapter will now discuss them separately, beginning with pets. The data presented in Part II yields several patterns with WDAS's pets. First, WDAS's pets often overlap with other character roles. For example, they often serve as sidekicks or minions. This is because they are often anthropomorphised. Second, whilst pets are almost-always anthropomorphised, they are often mute (67%). Generally, the more anthropomorphic a WDAS character is, the more central they are to the narrative's plot. This may be why pets are more anthropomorphised than working animals but less so than primary characters. Third, in many films, pets animals *want* to be pets rather than live in the wild or their natural habitat. WDAS's pets seem to dote on their owners, even when their owners are villainous. Fourth, cats and dogs are WDAS's most common pets (27% of the time). This means that WDAS's pet characters do somewhat reflect the reality of pet ownership. Fifth, most (69%) of WDAS's pets are mammals. This is probably because pets have to be species that humans like, and domesticated mammals usually score higher on the socio-zoological scale than species such as fish and reptiles do. Sixth, WDAS's pets tend to be associated with the locations they are based in. For example, *Lady and the Tramp* features dog breeds that are native to the UK, which is where the film is set. Thus, there is a reasonable amount of contextual realism to WDAS's pet characters.

As the data in Part II demonstrates, 57% of all WDAS films feature a human character with some kind of pet. In reality, pets are in danger of being mutilated, euthanized, caged, and so forth (*PETA* 2019e). Some of these harms have been selectively depicted in WDAS films, but there has been much romanticization of pet ownership too. To illustrate, *Bolt*, *Lady and the Tramp*, and *The Aristocats* all imply, or in some cases explicitly state, that being a human's pet is the best possible life for an animal. For example, in *Bolt*, both Bolt and Mittens desire a human owner rather than a life outdoors. Additionally, some harms that pets experience are depicted as comical rather than harmful. For instance, in *Pinocchio*, Cleo's goldfish bowl is turned black after being used to extinguish a fire naively started by Pinocchio. Subsequently, Cleo (who is a goldfish) is seen coughing at the surface of the water. However, this moment is designed to humorously convey Pinocchio's naivety, rather than the dangers of polluting a goldfish bowl; thus, the negligence displayed towards Cleo's well-being is eschewed.

As is the case with other forms of harm, WDAS often blames pets for their own misfortune. For example, in *The Fox and the Hound*, Tod (the pet fox) is released into the forest after repeatedly behaving in an uncivilized, non-pet-like, manner. Tod had been adopted by Widow Tweed as an infant and raised as a pet. The narrative implies that Tod's status as a pet is rescinded because of his un-domestic behaviour. For example, he chases chickens, which he is repeatedly warned not to do. Rather than suggesting that Widow Tweed is neglectful for abandoning Tod, the narrative is sympathetic towards her position. For example, sombre low-tempo instrumental music plays over the moment she abandons him in the forest and the build-up to it. Additionally, Widow Tweed is shown as physically distressed by the situation. She repeatedly shakes her head and cries as she leaves Tod in the forest alone. This is problematic because it suggests that Tweed is more harmed by the abandonment than Tod is. Tod does not cry as he is left alone, whereas Tweed cries as she drives off. As highlighted in Part I, animals become pets because their owner wants them, and not vice versa. Therefore, it is reasonable to expect humans to take responsibility for the welfare of their pets. Yet *The Fox and the Hound* offers more sympathy for Widow Tweed than Tod. By implying that disobedient pets deserve punishment, WDAS suggests that pets can be responsible for their own misfortune. As this book has demonstrated elsewhere, similar approaches can also be seen with other types of animal harm in WDAS films. For example, as Chap. 1 demonstrated, the farm animals in *Home on the Range* only faced harm *after* they left their dairy farm. Thus, their later misfortunate was depicted as a result of their own choices.

Similar to WDAS's portrayal of other types of animal harm, pets that face mistreatment or harm often escape or manage to improve their situation. For example, in *Peter Pan*, the Darling family have a beloved pet dog called Nana. At the beginning of the narrative, Nana is forced to sleep outdoors in a dog kennel by George Darling. Nana is not happy with the situation; she frowns and walks limply as she is dragged outside by George. However, a few hours later, George has a change of heart and allows Nana back inside for the night. Therefore, her mistreatment is mild and only temporary. Similarly, stray animals usually manage to find loving homes in WDAS films. For example, Tramp (*Lady and the Tramp*), Mittens (*Bolt*), and Thomas O'Malley (*The Aristocats*) are all stray animals that find permanent loving homes at the end of their respective narratives. In another example, during the birth of the puppies in *Dalmatians*, one of the puppies appears to be stillborn. While "dead", the puppy is covered with a blanket. Upon seeing this, Roger (the owner of the Dalmatians) rubs the puppy gently until it comes to life. Thus, in some cases, humans can improve, and even save, their pets' lives.

Similarly, some potentially harmful ways of treating pets, such as spoiling them, are depicted as acts of love and care in WDAS films. In fact, it is often implied that the owners who spoil their pets care more about their pets than those who do not. For example, in *Oliver & Company*, Jenny demonstrates her love and affection towards her pets by offering them expensive luxury accessories and large amounts of food. It is notable that the pets spoiled most frequently are WDAS's villainous pets, which are often showered with material possessions by their owners. Indeed, some of WDAS's villains appear to treat their pets exceptionally well. One of the most pampered pets is Percy, the pet of Ratcliffe (the main antagonist) in *Pocahontas*, for example.

While some of the harmful aspects of pet ownership have been depicted or acknowledged, others have not. The practices that have not been depicted, or have only been depicted once, are the ones that are the most controversial in reality. For example, the euthanasia of homeless pets has only been depicted once (*Lady and the Tramp*), and it is depicted as terrifying. Tail docking, ear cropping, and similar harmful practices have never been depicted or referenced, even though they are common practices in reality (Sinmez et al. 2017: 431–437). De-clawing has been referenced once (*Bolt*), and it is depicted as being unnecessary and cruel. Towards the end of *Bolt*, Mittens (the cat) confides in Bolt (the dog) that her previous owners had de-clawed her. The process of de-clawing is not shown, but Mittens is clearly upset and embarrassed by her lack of claws. She blurts out that she is declawed whilst angrily telling Bolt why she distrusts humans. Therefore, this scene implies that de-clawing is cruel and harmful to cats. Since many of these pet-keeping practices are socially-unacceptable, they are more challenging to romanticize and minimize, which is likely why WDAS has mostly avoided them. This is similar to the way that WDAS has avoided the more controversial side of farming, such as the production of foie gras and veal, as Chap. 1 highlighted. Additionally, *Lady and the Tramp*, *Dalmatians*, and *Aristocats* all feature pets with offspring that they are allowed to keep. In none of these three examples are any of the infants removed from their parents, nor is this even suggested. In fact, in *Dalmatians*, the dog-owners refuse to sell their many puppies even though it is implied that they are struggling financially. In fact, they later agree to give homes to even more puppies despite their financial woes. Despite this, it is very common for pets to have their offspring removed in reality (for example: *The Kennel Club* 2019b). Thus, some situations depict the romantic opposite of pet-keeping.

Given the prevalence of pets in WDAS films, it is perhaps unusual that very few pet shops, shelters, and so forth are depicted. Additionally, WDAS has never depicted a veterinary hospital or similar. On the few occasions that pet shops have been depicted, they have been presented in a neutral or positive manner. For example, animals for sale in pet shops are usually portrayed as happy with their situation. To illustrate, in *Lady and the Tramp*, the Cocker Spaniel puppies in the pet shop window are grinning and wagging their tails. Additionally, the shops themselves are clean and spacious. Thus, the more objectionable side of these locations has never been depicted. This will be further discussed in Part IV with *Lady and the Tramp*. In contrast, shelters/pounds have been depicted more negatively but also rarely. For example, in *Lady and the Tramp*, a dog is euthanized in a pound. In *Bolt*, Mittens and Bolt are caught and kept in a shelter for a short while. The cages they are held in are depicted as small and uncomfortable. These small dark cages contrast with the vast outdoor locations where Bolt and Mittens were previously roaming. However, every primary animal character that is taken to a shelter in a WDAS film manages to escape. This suggests that shelters are harmful, uncomfortable locations, but also that they are escapable. This is both an acknowledgement of the unfair treatment pets can also experience, but it is also a romanticization of reality. In reality, animals in shelters, pounds, and so forth, have an extremely low chance of escape.

As the previous paragraphs highlight, WDAS has occasionally depicted direct harm towards pet animals. However, as with the types of harm highlighted and discussed in the previous chapters, WDAS has minimized, romanticized, and attenuated some of these issues. Additionally, pets that face harm are usually able to escape their mistreatment and find a better life, which is another way in which the real issues some pets experience are negated.

WDAS's pet characters can be divided into two categories: pets as protagonists and pets as supporting characters. These different types of pet face different harms and forms of discrimination. For example, the only pets to have died have been villainous secondary pets. Therefore, this chapter will now discuss pets as protagonists and pets as secondary characters separately.

A protagonist pet is an animal character that is the main character of their narrative, but also has a human owner (who is usually a supporting character). Pet protagonists can be seen in *Lady and the Tramp*, *The Aristocats*, and *Bolt*, for example. While there are several villainous pets in WDAS films, none of them are main characters. Thus, all of WDAS's pet protagonists are pro-social characters. Films that feature pet protagonists usually have human villains. For example, the villain in *The Aristocats* is Edgar Balthazar, a human, even though the narrative is centred around cats. Pet protagonists are much more independent and anthropomorphised than secondary pets. For example, they are all able to speak. In contrast, pets that are secondary characters are usually mute. However, pet protagonists usually only speak to other animals and rarely to humans. Despite being more anthropomorphised than secondary pets, pet protagonists are never heavily-anthropomorphised in the same way that non-pet animal protagonists, such as Mickey Mouse, are. For example, WDAS's pet protagonists rarely wear clothing, walk upright, and so forth. They always maintain some of their non-human qualities, such as walking on all-fours. Classic Disney animators, Thomas and Johnston (1981) claim that:

> If an animal in a film is wearing any kind of costume, he can be handled with human attributes and the audience will accept him. In contrast, if an animal in his natural fur should suddenly stand up and start gesticulating, the viewers will feel uneasy. Put a cap on him, or a tie, and he can swagger around, gesturing and pointing like any ham actor. (Thomas and Johnston 1981: 331)

This suggests that the reason pets often retain many of their animal-like qualities is because of their lack of clothing. However, this lack of clothing is necessary for the realism of these characters.

WDAS's secondary pets are generally less-anthropomorphised than WDAS's protagonist pets. This is evident in several ways. First, they are usually mute and can only produce animal sounds, even though the other animal characters in their diegetic world can often speak. For example, in *Cinderella*, Lucifer (the pet cat) cannot speak, but the mice can. Second, secondary pets rarely wear much clothing. In fact, they are often "naked", i.e. not wearing any human clothing at all. Third, they always seem to keep some non-human traits, such as walking on all-fours. They are not fully-anthropomorphised like Goofy the dog is, for example. To illustrate, in *Pinocchio*, Figaro (Geppetto's cat) is mute, but Gideon (Honest John's sidekick cat) wears a full outfit. This is perhaps because pets need to be less-developed than the main character they are associated with to avoid upstaging them (Simpson 2001: 39). However, this point evidently does not apply to the other animal characters in the secondary pet's diegetic world. As the quote from Thomas and Johnston in the previous paragraph highlights, "naked" animals cannot be too heavily-anthropomorphised, or they become uncanny.

Protagonists and antagonists need to have something distinguishing about their character or appearance to make them memorable, but this is not usually the case for the pets of these characters, which are usually less-developed, detailed, and unique. The normalness of secondary pets often complements the main character by making them look more beautiful or special, or, in the case of antagonistic pets, uglier or more disgusting. This lack of detail further implies that pets are subordinate to their owner. To illustrate, WDAS's human princesses are always very detailed in appearance; however, their pets are often designed with far fewer distinguishing details. This subservience is furthered through the pet's lack of voice, which is very common with WDAS's secondary pets, even though they are often anthropomorphised. By characterizing pets with non-verbal communication, WDAS implies that these characters are less important to the narrative. This lack of voice also stops the character from voicing any discomfort or unhappiness that they may face. In reality, animals cannot speak; however, in WDAS films, they often can, especially when they are supporting characters. Thus, the fact that WDAS has an entire category of animal characters that usually cannot speak suggests that there is a reason these characters do not speak. That reason is because they are pets, and their human owner is the more important character. As well as being lower-status, pet characters are always physically smaller than the human they are associated with. For example, in *Tangled*, Pascale often sits on Rapunzel's shoulder. His diminutive size seems to serve as a metaphor for the difference in character status between the two, i.e. that pets usually have a smaller, less-important, role in the narrative. This contrasts with pets as protagonists, which are often larger pets. To illustrate, in *Dalmatians*, the Dalmatians are smaller than their owner, as pets usually are, yet they are much larger than almost-all of WDAS's secondary pets.

WDAS's secondary pets fulfil various narrative functions, such as: comedy, friendship, rescue, and so forth. Their role depends on the type of story they exist in, and the type of character they are associated with. For example, villainous pets always have villainous owners, and small male animals often accompany female princesses. Secondary pets often fill the void of loneliness for humans that are alone due to personal tragedy (Mollet 2013: 109–124). This can be clearly seen in *The Rescuers* and *Tangled*, both of which feature female human characters that have been socially isolated from other humans. These narratives imply that this character only has a pet because they struggle to form relationships with humans. This is problematic because it implies that the only purpose of these pets is to alleviate the loneliness of humans. Additionally, the animal's own desires are rarely mentioned in these texts, only the human character's wishes. Therefore, these films imply that pets are accessories to humans, rather than individuals worthy of their own characterization and story.

Every pet owned by a human antagonist is villainous. WDAS's villainous pets differ from non-villainous pets in several ways. First, the pets of villains tend to be less developed, or more minor, characters than the pets of protagonist characters are. For example, they are more likely to be mute than non-villainous pets are. Second, in many cases, villains abandon their pet, or vice-versa, by the end of the text. For example, Percy (Ratcliffe's Pug in *Pocahontas*) stays with Pocahontas in America, and Joanna waves off McLeach as he falls to his implied (off-screen) death in *The Rescuers Down Under*. This type of ending does not happen with the pets of pro-social characters. Therefore, the relationship between a villain and their pet is evidently less loyal than the relationship between pro-social owners and their pets. Third, a common occurrence with WDAS's villainous pets is that they often die or face severe punishment at the end of their film. For example, Diablo (*Sleeping Beauty*) is turned into stone, and Iago (*Aladdin*) is trapped in a lamp for 10,000 years. In contrast, the pets of protagonists never die or face severe harm. Therefore, it is implied that it is acceptable for villainous animals to die or face harm. As a result, the human characters who harm pets are not necessarily villains. Some of WDAS's pro-social human characters, i.e. those who typically demonstrate kind and caring behaviour, have exhibited cruelty towards pet animals. For example, in *Sleeping Beauty*, Diablo (Maleficent's pet raven) is turned into stone by Merryweather, one of the film's charming fairy godmothers. As Chap. 2 demonstrated, any harms experienced by villainous animals (such as when the hunting dogs in *Bambi* fall off a cliff) are depicted as deserved rather than cruel. Fourth, previous research has found that certain types of villains are often associated with certain colours, themes, or even animal species. For example, female villains are often associated with lower-ranked species of animals: Medusa with crocodilians, Maleficent with a raven, and so forth (Bowman 2011: 93). In contrast, male villains tend to have higher-ranked species of pet. To illustrate, Jafar (*Aladdin*) has a parrot, and Sykes (*Oliver & Company*) has two Dobermans. This implies that certain colours and species of animals are associated with villainous characters. However, this colour-scheme is problematic because it suggests that black animals are evil, an association that has affected real animals negatively. For example, it has been found that black cats are less-likely to be adopted from shelters (Kogan 2013:18–22).

WDAS's Working Animals[5]

As is clear from this text's data, working animals are a significant part of WDAS's cast of characters. They are included in 54% of WDAS films, which makes them almost as common as pets. WDAS's working animals

[5] The author of this book also authored a blog post for *The Society of Animation Studies*, which discusses similar ideas to those raised here. The blog post can be found at: Stanton 2019.

seem to be realistic when compared to real working animals. For example, all of WDAS's working animals are mammals, which is also usually the case in reality (*SPANA* 2019a). Also similar to reality, the welfare of working animals is rarely portrayed as important in WDAS films. In most WDAS films, working animals exist in the background of the text as genderless, nameless, non-anthropomorphised characters.

Horses occupy a unique role in human culture. Like dogs and cats, they have lived alongside humans for thousands of years, yet unlike dogs and cats, they have remained outdoors (*Blue Cross* 2019). Unlike dogs, which also have a long history working alongside humans, horses rarely fall into the pet role. They almost-always stay as working animals and are usually killed when no longer useful (Surendra 2019). The reason why working animals like horses are rarely considered pets is likely because of their large size. Humans prefer animals smaller than themselves, such as cats, or much larger, such as elephants (MacClellan 2013: 57–68). This is likely to be one of the key reasons why most working animals, such as horses, are rarely seen as pets. A significant number (65%) of WDAS's working animals are horses. In fact, horses are the second most commonly depicted species across all of the fifty-six WDAS films in this study. However, despite their prevalence, horses are often non-anthropomorphised, nameless, genderless, and without individual personalities. This is unusual because WDAS typically anthropomorphises and individualizes their animal characters, as was demonstrated earlier with pets. WDAS's most notable characters are their heavily-anthropomorphised, individualized, named ones, such as Mickey Mouse, Simba, and Jiminy Cricket. However, animals are only given names when they are special to humans (Borkfelt 2011: 116–125). Therefore, the fact that the majority of WDAS's horses are nameless suggests that WDAS does not deem horses to be special or unique animals. Moreover, very few of WDAS's horses have a clear gender. The lack of gender is notable because WDAS films are infamous for their reliance and reinforcement of gender stereotypes, even with animal characters. To be optimistic, WDAS's lack of gender stereotypes with horses could be seen as progressive rather than unfair. However, given that gender is a significant part of the personality of many of WDAS's animal characters, it seems more likely that this lack of gender is because these characters lack detail. Thus, their lack of gender does not liberate these animals, it objectifies them.

Despite being WDAS's second-most commonly-depicted species, horses have never been the main character of any WDAS film. They mostly exist as background characters to provide transportation for human characters. Since many WDAS films are set before the Industrial Revolution, the inclusion of horses for transportation is necessary for historical realism. In no WDAS film does a horse exist solely for companionship; their primary purpose is always to transport humans or loads. Moreover, unlike pets, horses do not usually have personalities that echo their human owner's personality. For example, human villains do not usually have antagonistic horses. Thus, working animals imply much less about the human they are associated with than pets do. These points suggest that WDAS depicts horses as objects rather than sentient, individual, animals. Their value is solely based on their ability to transport humans rather than their potential for companionship.

Further to this, working animals sometimes face direct harm and neglect in WDAS films, yet their narratives encourage little sympathy for their pain. For example, in *Make Mine Music*, two non-anthropomorphised cart horses are whipped to instruct them to move. In another example, the non-anthropomorphised donkeys that transport Pinocchio to "Pleasure Island" in *Pinocchio* are repeatedly whipped and have rocks catapulted at them. However, because the animals in both examples are not individualized or anthropomorphised, their mistreatment is less likely to elicit sympathy. Certainly, in neither example does the narrative encourage sympathy when these animals are harmed. For example, there is no sombre music or pained reaction from other characters, which are common when an anthropomorphised animal is harmed or dies, such as after the death of Bambi's mother. This lack of pause for the harms inflicted upon working animals suggests that working animals do not feel pain, or perhaps that the human need for animal labour is prioritized over the animal's suffering. It also further supports the notion that WDAS's working animals are depicted as objects rather than sentient animals.

The ethics of making animals work have largely gone unquestioned in WDAS films, which was also the case for farmed animals as Chap. 1

demonstrated. Furthermore, since most of WDAS's working animals are non-anthropomorphised, their happiness, or unhappiness, is not evident. One of the only films that questions the ethics of making animals work is *The Fox and the Hound*, in which Copper (a dog) refuses to fulfil his role as a hunting dog after befriending a local fox. This situation suggests that working is a choice for Copper. Despite his training, Copper refuses to harm the fox, and Amos (his owner) accepts Copper's choice without punishing him. In reality, working animals have no choice over the job assigned to them. They are trained to perform jobs, and if they do not do so, they are often punished or even killed (for example: Barnett 2006). The fact that this rebellion happens with a dog, rather than a horse is significant. Horses are much more common as working animals, yet they have never been depicted as seriously rebelling against their role. This suggests that WDAS's working dogs are characterized as having greater sentience and free will than horses. Rebellion is also evident with some other species of working animal, albeit to a lesser extent. For example, in *Snow White*, the cart-pulling deer kicks Sleepy (one of the dwarves) after he mistakenly hits the deer with a stick. This implies that the deer is in control of the situation and able to reject any mistreatment, which is another romanticization of the reality working animals experience. However, there is one film which implies that working animals have challenging and depressing lives. In *Pinocchio*, various boys (including Pinocchio) are tricked into going to "Pleasure Island". Once there, they are transformed into mute donkeys and forced into small crates. The crates are labelled with "sold to the salt mine" and similar. Thus, the metamorphosed donkeys are almost-certainly going to be forced into working, which distresses them. Therefore, WDAS has fleetingly acknowledged the cruelty of forcing animals into work, but in a way that centres the feelings and fears of humans, rather than working animals.

To conclude Parts II and III, it seems clear that even though pets and working animals are common characters in WDAS films, they have been characterized very differently. WDAS's pets are usually named, anthropomorphised, and individualized, but they are often mute. In contrast, WDAS's working animals are usually non-anthropomorphised, genderless, nameless, and without distinguishing characteristics. Moreover, unlike pets, working animals do not usually further characterize the human characters they exist alongside, which pets do. Thus, WDAS's pet characters have been much more detailed and individualized than WDAS's working animals have been.

There is some acknowledgement of the mistreatment and harm pets and working animals can experience in WDAS films. However, the most controversial forms of harming pets and working animals have not yet been depicted, which is consistent with WDAS's portrayal of other forms of animal harm. For example, in regards to pets, euthanasia and declawing have both been depicted once, but castration and puppy farming have never been. The exception to this point is antagonistic pets. In many cases, villainous pets are severely harmed or even killed in WDAS films, which is depicted as deserved rather than cruel. This is similar to how WDAS depicted the hunting of antagonistic animals as justifiable, which was highlighted in Chap. 2. The issues working animals experience have mostly been focussed upon when they involve dogs or humans, i.e. a higher-order species. Moreover, WDAS has never depicted a working animal being killed for rebelling against their assigned job, which is common in reality. However, as Part I demonstrated, the lack of attention given to WDAS's working animals may be reflective of reality since working animals are often metaphorically-objectified in real life, while pets are not. This chapter will now explore some of these points alongside *Lady and the Tramp*, a WDAS film that focusses on pets but also features working animals.

Part IV: Pets, Working Animals, and *Lady and the Tramp*

Lady and the Tramp (1955) was released in 1955, during WDAS's "Silver Age".[6] It was adapted from two short stories.[7] As highlighted in the previous chapter with *Dalmatians,* WDAS often removes or attenuates animal harm during their text-to-film adaptation process. However, *Lady and the Tramp* is one of the few WDAS films that *adds* direct harm towards animals during its adaptation process. *Lady and the Tramp* includes an animal pound, euthanasia, a muzzle, neglect, and so forth. However, from this information it should not be assumed that WDAS was attempting to break boundaries here. The inclusion of animal harm serves a vital function to the expanded storyline devised by WDAS, which will be further detailed in this section.

As with WDAS's other early animal-focussed films, such as *Bambi* and *Dumbo*, many of the dog characters in *Lady and the Tramp* were animated directly from live animals (*American Film Institute* 2017). For example, "Lady" was modelled from the pet Cocker Spaniel of the voice actor for Aunt Sarah (*American Film Institute* 2017). However, there is no evidence that the horses were animated from live horses, which is in contrast to the detailed dog characters. While horses are a large species, WDAS is evidenced to have directly animated from other large species previously. For example, when producing *Dumbo*, WDAS's artists animated from live

[6] Disney's "Silver Age" (1950–1967) was an era that replicated many of the well-loved trends established during Disney's "Golden Age" (1937–42) but abandoned during Disney's "Wartime Era" (1943–9). Disney's "Silver Age" returned to using detailed backgrounds and soft colours, techniques previously found in the "Golden Age". During this time, Disney also began to invest in more complex characters alongside their "sentimental modernism" (Watts 1995: 95).

[7] The idea for *Lady and the Tramp* initially came from Joe Grant, one of Disney's own in-house artists and writers, in 1937. Grant's story was based upon his experience with his own pet Springer Spaniel, Lady, which had been neglected after the birth of Grant's first baby. Walt liked Grant's sketches and asked Grant to expand the idea into a storyboard. However, once story-boarded, Walt did not like the full narrative, so the idea was abandoned. A few years later, Walt bought the rights to the illustrated short story *Happy Dan, the Whistling Dog* by Ward Greene. Walt believed that the two dog-focussed short stories could be combined into one to create a feature length film (Beck 2005: 136–137). This combination became *Lady and the Tramp*, and production began a few years later. The delay between finding the two stories and animation was primarily because of World War Two. During the Second World War, the Disney studios spent much of their time and resources making propaganda animations (Teurlay 2014).

elephants, which are generally much larger than horses (Pallant 2011: 47). Thus, the reason WDAS did not animate directly from live horses is likely because of speciesism rather than practicality. It is also well-documented that the animators had a miniature model of Lady's home that they used to animate the film from a dog's point of view (*American Film Institute* 2017). This is why the faces of the human characters are not usually seen. This further suggests that WDAS prioritized the dogs over the other species in the film. Indeed, these speciesist attitudes are then reflected throughout the film, especially through its characterization of pets and working animals.

Lady and the Tramp centres around the issue of pet-ownership, and the problems it can cause for animals and humans. The main protagonist is Lady, a female Cocker-Spaniel who belongs to a young middle-class couple. When Lady is first introduced, she is a gift-wrapped puppy in a hat box.[8] Lady is boxed because she is being given to Darling as a Christmas present from Jim Dear.[9] This scene is problematic because it metaphorically objectifies pets, yet this objectification is masked behind romance. This scene, in which a young married couple celebrate Christmas together, has a romantic atmosphere. The scene opens with a shot of a small, peaceful, village. Snow falls gently over the large houses, making it clear that it is winter. The next shot is inside the Darling's home, which is tastefully decorated for Christmas. This romantic, peaceful, festive, atmosphere distracts from the ethical issues this scene has. Lady is presented as a wrapped Christmas gift, similar to how objects are gifted. Additionally, her box has no holes, which would be vital to the welfare of a live animal in this situation. Thus, even though the film's depictions of dogs are positive, it begins by metaphorically objectifying them. As the film progresses, Lady is established as an independent character and thus not metaphorically objectified further. However, this opening shot establishes her place as a pet dog. It makes it clear that Lady is a human's pet and thus *belongs* to humans.

[8] This scene was famously based upon a real moment in Walt's life when he gifted a puppy to Lillian (his wife) in a hat box (*American Film Institute* 2017).

[9] Perhaps because the film is from a dog's viewpoint, most of the human characters do not have realistic names. Lady refers to her owners as "Jim Dear" and "Darling" throughout the text, and their real names are never given (*IMDB* 2016).

Lady's background, such as her mother and littermates, is not mentioned. However, the fact that she is in a box and being gifted suggests that she was purchased. This implies that it is ethical, and even romantic, to buy puppies as Christmas presents. As Part I of this chapter evidenced, Disney films significantly influence the breeds of dogs subsequently sold in reality. Therefore, it seems reasonable to suggest that this influence could also affect how and when dogs are sold. *Lady and the Tramp* was released in 1955, before animal welfare charities urged people not to buy dogs as Christmas presents (*Dogs Trust* 2018). It was in 1978 that Dogs Trust [sic] (which at the time was named the National Canine Defence League) first ran their influential "A dog is for life, not just for Christmas" campaign. This campaign encouraged people not to buy dogs impulsively at Christmas time or to gift them as Christmas presents. This was because animal shelters noticed a trend in dogs being adopted before Christmas, and then returned to shelters in January–March (*Dogs Trust* 2018). Thus, at the time of the film's release, the act of gifting a puppy could have been seen as romantic rather than harmful. Yet despite this, the scene is still problematic from an animal welfare perspective because it metaphorically objectifies animals.

On her first night as a pet, Lady is placed into a small basket with a blanket and pillow. The basket looks like it is designed for a human baby rather than a puppy. Additionally, Lady is placed on her back, again as if she is a human baby, not a puppy. Lady smiles widely during this moment, suggesting that she is comfortable in this human-like, rather than dog-like, sleeping position. By depicting Lady as a small puppy, sleeping like a human baby, WDAS makes Lady appear vulnerable. Lady spends most of the film as an adult dog, but her introduction as a needy, vulnerable, puppy encourages nurturing feelings from the audience. This is similar to the care-giving reaction that occurs when audiences see a neotenous character (Lamarre 2011: 124). However, given that Lady was metaphorically-objectified in the previous scene (by being gifted as a Christmas present), this scene is perhaps an improvement from an animal welfare perspective. It establishes that Lady is not an object; she is a puppy with similar needs to a human baby.

After Lady's owners leave her alone in her basket downstairs, she cries and whines. However, she is crying because she has been separated from her owners, not because she misses her own mother, or because of her human-like sleeping conditions. Once she escapes from the downstairs room, she immediately makes her way upstairs and into her owner's bed, where she is then depicted as comfortable and happy. This is problematic because it suggests that humans are more important to puppies than their own canine family. The film then fast-forwards to Lady at six-months old, and she is still sleeping in her owner's bed. Therefore, Lady was able to permanently escape a situation she disliked with relative ease. Whilst Lady was unhappy with being isolated, this situation could not be considered harmful when studied alongside some of the common issues pets experience in reality, such as being permanently caged. This is another example of WDAS questioning simple, often unharmful, situations, rather than more challenging problems, such as the forced separation of puppies from their mother.

Once Darling and Jim Dear learn that they are expecting a baby, they become less considerate and attentive towards Lady. For example, Jim Dear refers to Lady as "that dog", which greatly upsets Lady. This is problematic because a real dog is unlikely to be offended by insensitive words or phrases. Within *Lady and the Tramp*, the pet animals speak to each other and understand English; however, they do not speak directly to the human characters, and it seems that the humans do not know that their pets can understand them. Thus, it would appear that Jim Dear does not know that his language offends Lady. Despite this, Jim's language towards Lady is still undignified, whether she can understand it or not. It suggests that Jim lacks respect for Lady. Lady then reveals to the other dogs that Darling hit her after she misbehaved. However, Lady adds that the slap did not hurt. In fact, Lady explicitly states that the insensitive words said by Jim Dear hurt her more than the physical violence from Darling did. These two instances, the slap and Jim's curt words, highlight that Lady is being excluded from the familial in-group that she believed she previously belonged to. However, the issue with this scene is that real dogs are unlikely to be harmed by curt words and are more likely to be harmed by physical violence. Thus, *Lady and the Tramp* creates anthropocentric problems that do not exist for pet dogs rather than depicting the real problems that pets can experience. Given the effect that Disney films have had upon real pets, this is problematic. Research suggests that depictions of pets in cultural representations can influence how people treat animals in reality. Thus, by suggesting that insensitive words can hurt dogs more than physical harm, Disney could be influencing how people treat their dogs in reality. If Disney implies that words can hurt dogs more than violence, this could cause people to minimize violence towards pets in reality.

In the middle of the film, Lady is caught by the dog catcher and taken to the dog pound after wandering the streets with Tramp. In the dog pound, Lady is clearly more neotenous, better spoken, and better behaved than the homeless dogs. Lady speaks with an upper-class Received Pronunciation British accent, which contrasts with most of the other dogs in the pound. For example, the British Bulldog (named Bull) speaks in a cockney accent, suggesting that he is more working-class than Lady is. The other dogs refer to Lady as "Miss Park Avenue" after sensing that she is someone's pet rather than a stray like them. Lady was likely designed with civilized behaviour and an attractive appearance to make her instinctively more-likeable than the other dog characters. Humans prefer animals with similar appearance and behaviour to themselves, which is why WDAS's animal protagonists are normally their most human-like characters in both behaviour and appearance (Westbury and Neumann 2008: 66–74). This instinctively encourages sympathy for Lady's plight, much more so than the other dogs, who behave in less-civilized ways. For example, Bull drools as he speaks, which makes his behaviour animalistic. It is implied that the other dogs in the pound are likely to be euthanized if they do not find homes, but their fate is not returned to, only Lady's is.[10] Thus, like WDAS's other animal-centred films, only the welfare of specific animals (which are usually the most anthropomorphised and neotenous) is implied to be important. The film cannot follow the life of every animal character. However, it is clear that the other dog characters in this film have more challenging and less-hopeful lives than Lady. Therefore, WDAS is again only addressing simple, easily-resolved, issues that animals experience, rather than the darker, more hopeless, issues, which are

[10] The fate of these dogs is not returned to in *Lady and the Tramp*; however, two of the stray dogs (Peg and Bull) have a cameo appearance six years later in 1961's *One Hundred and One Dalmatians*. This suggests that they are re-homed or similar (*Animation Source* 2018).

much more challenging to romanticize. This scene also demonstrates how Singer's argument about personhood can be applied to animals. The dogs in the pound have lost some of their individuality and thus personhood because they do not have families; their diminished state of personhood makes their lives appear less-valuable than Lady's, which adds to the tone of despair surrounding these characters.

The other dog protagonist is Tramp, who initially contrasts greatly with Lady in both appearance and behaviour. To illustrate, he is less neotenous and human-like than her. For example, in the scene before Lady is sent to the pound, Tramp wants to chase chickens, but Lady does not because she is concerned that they will hurt the chickens if they do. Chasing chickens is a behaviour that is somewhat natural to dogs; therefore, the fact that Lady does not want to do it suggests that she no longer has her natural dog instincts, which Trampdoes (Willis and Ludlow 2015: 18, 39). While Tramp appears to be a stray dog, he claims to have a different home for every night of the week. Certainly, he has no problem sourcing food or shelter. This is another example of WDAS romanticizing the common problems some animals experience. Stray dogs are likely to suffer from hunger, cold weather, and so forth (Mullins 2018). However, none of these issues seem to affect Tramp. For example, Tramp is twice shown visiting an Italian restaurant and being swiftly offered large plates of food by the obliging waiters. Thus, hunger and sourcing food are not issues that affect Tramp. Additionally, Tramp is never portrayed as being cold or without adequate shelter. When Lady spends the night with Tramp outdoors, they sleep in a peaceful park and show no signs of being cold or uncomfortable. In fact, Tramp repeatedly states that he enjoys living outdoors. Tramp's past is not directly mentioned; however, it is implied that Tramp was abandoned by his previous owners. Upon meeting Lady and hearing of the neglect she is experiencing due to Darling's pregnancy, Tramp tells Lady that it is common for dogs to be abandoned once their owners have a baby. He impersonates human mothers with an exaggerated screechy voice during this scene:

Tramp: "Put that dog out! He'll get fleas all over the baby". You start barking at some strange mutt. "Stop that racket! You'll wake the baby".

The sentences in quotation marks are spoken with an impersonated screechy female voice by Tramp. This screechy exaggeration in Tramp's voice makes the scene comical rather than depressing. Tramp seems to be speaking from experience, which suggests that he was abandoned. Tramp's implied abandonment is a depressing problem that affects many dogs in reality (*PETA* 2018a). However, rather than depicting this issue as miserable, WDAS opted to make it comical. Thus, this is another example of WDAS joking about, and thus minimizing, the real, and very common, problems that affect pet animals. Of course, as the previous chapter demonstrated, WDAS minimized and joked about the fur industry with *Dalmatians*. However, after the release of *Dalmatians*, fur clothing became much less popular; thus, WDAS's comical approach (albeit unrealistic) helped change attitudes towards the fur industry. Yet in *Lady and the Tramp*, this comical approach does not benefit pet animals, and it is for the same reasons that *Home on the Range* did not benefit farm animals. By implying that abandoning pets can be comical, WDAS portrays this issue as socially-acceptable. Similarly, in *Home on the Range*, WDAS masked the problems of the dairy industry behind happy farm animals and jokes. In *Dalmatians*, even though the film joked about the fur industry, the fur industry was still depicted unfavourably. This is why the comedy utilized in *Dalmatians* is not problematic, but the comedy in *Lady and the Tramp* and *Home on the Range* is.

One of the film's most famous aspects is the love story between Lady and Tramp. Lady, the upper-class pure-bred house dog, falls in love with Tramp, an "Average Joe" street dog (Spector 1998: 46). The film ends with Lady and Tramp living at Lady's home together with their new-born puppies. This type of ending is common in WDAS's love stories involving animals. WDAS's animal romances usually end with offspring, whereas WDAS's human romances often end in marriage. Of course, in reality, dog breeds like Lady usually have their mate chosen for them by humans (for example: *The Kennel Club* 2019a). Despite being a famous filmic animal romance, the love story between Lady and Tramp is evident solely from their human-like behaviour. To illustrate, the dogs famously eat spaghetti at a restaurant table together. They also intentionally place their paws and sign their initials in wet cement. Their love is not evident from dog-like behaviour. For example, they do not sniff and lick each other, which is how real dogs demonstrate affection towards each other (Hoffman and Ackerman 1998: 161). Therefore, the film anthropomorphises the relationships of dogs. Films that feature pro-social dog characters influence the dogs that are bought in reality. However, it has been found that many dog owners are often surprised to learn that their new pets exhibit behaviour far-removed from their romantic anthropomorphised Disney portrayal (Henderson and Anderson 2005: 297). Therefore, Disney's romantic anthropomorphised portrayal of dogs in films such as *Lady and the Tramp* is unlikely to benefit animals in reality, quite the opposite.

Lady and the Tramp has several villainous characters. Two of the villains are Si and Am, two identical Siamese pet cats that belong to Aunt Sarah. Aunt Sarah brings them to Lady's house and lets them roam free, which results in chaos. Si and Am intentionally harass Lady, the pet bird, and the pet fish. After causing destruction, they manipulatively portray themselves as the victims to Aunt Sarah, which results in Lady being forced to wear a muzzle. Cats are often viewed as a villainous species in wider culture (Peterson and Farrington 2007: 24). Therefore, it is unsurprising that this is how they are commonly depicted in WDAS films, such as *Lady and the Tramp*. The problem with Si and Am is that they cause many of the problems Lady subsequently experiences, such as wearing a muzzle and then ending up in a dog pound. Thus, this is another instance in which animals are to blame for the problems that they, or other animals, experience. *Lady and the Tramp* is about pet animals, yet half of the villains in this text are other animals, not humans. As highlighted in Part III, it is common for WDAS's human villains to have a villainous pet that causes problems for pro-social characters. For example, in *Cinderella*, Lucifer the cat (Lady Tremaine's pet) repeatedly harms the mice. Yet these villainous pets are problematic because they blame the mistreatment of pets on other animals. The problems pet animals experience in reality are solely because of humans not other animals.

Lady and the Tramp is one of just three WDAS films to feature a pound/shelter. The dog pound is the most miserable-looking location in the film. It is a run-down dark building surrounded by barbed wire, dark clouds, and barren land. This dark location contrasts with Lady's bright, colourful, spacious, house. In the pound, the dogs are locked in bare cages with just bowls of water and some straw. The first shot inside of the pound depicts several dogs crying, which implies a mood of despair. The bars of the cages are cast onto the dogs, making them look striped, as if they are wearing prisoner uniforms. The dogs are introduced through a harmonious, melodic, whine. After the music stops, it is revealed that the dogs are crying together in order to cover the sound of an escape tunnel that the Dachshund is digging. This is another example of WDAS making light of quite a serious situation. This escape tunnel implies that these dogs have a fair chance at escaping from the pound, which in reality, dogs in pounds do not. However, given the wider context of the film, this chance of escape is necessary as it adds hope to a situation that would otherwise be very depressing. It becomes clear soon after that dogs are being euthanized in this pound. If *Lady and the Tramp* offered no optimism for the caged dogs, it would not be as engaging to watch.

The dog pound scene is notable for containing WDAS's only depiction of euthanasia. The euthanasia is not explicitly shown, but it is suggested through dark shadows and soft, solemn, instrumental, low-tempo music. The dog that is euthanized is never fully shown, nor does it speak. It is only ever shown as a shadow walking alongside a human figure. The dog walks with its ears high, tail upright, and tongue out. Throughout the film it is implied that dogs are more aware of their surroundings than humans give them credit for. However, in this scene, the happiness of the shadowed dog, which is suggested through body language, implies that it is unaware of its morbid fate. The naivety of this one dog makes the situation seem more harmful. Because the dog is seemingly unaware of its fate, it does not attempt to escape, which the other dogs do. The shadowed dog is taken into a dark room at the back of the pound, which has a sign reading "Keep out". The other dogs are clearly aware of what will happen to the shadowed dog, and they explicitly state this. This suggestion of euthanasia makes Lady's situation much more serious than previously. Therefore, the purpose of this scene is to suggest that Lady could be killed if she remains in the pound. Thus, this scene is dramatic because it suggests Lady's potential fate, rather than because an un-characterized dog has been killed.

Lady and the Tramp also features a pet shop, which is shown twice. In the pet shop, the anthropomorphised animals for sale look happy with their situation. For example, when the shop is first depicted, there are some Cocker Spaniel puppies in a clean, cageless window display. They wag their tails happily as Tramp approaches the window to greet them. There is no adult dog, i.e. mother, present during this scene. This suggests that infant animals do not need their mothers to be happy. As highlighted earlier, this was also how Lady was depicted as a puppy: motherless yet happy. Therefore, this is another example of WDAS romanticizing, and thus ignoring, the ethically-challenging areas of pet ownership. However, this romantic pet shop is necessary to the film because it suggests that Lady was adopted from a pet shop that treated her well. This again distracts from the wider ethics of "buying" pet animals, a practice often criticized by animal welfare organizations.

As with many other WDAS films that focus on animals, *Lady and the Tramp* is speciesist. Both Lady and Tramp are shown eating meat and harming other animals. For instance, Tramp takes much pleasure is chasing a group of terrified non-anthropomorphised chickens. Tramp also suggests that the hyena in the zoo needs a muzzle after it laughs manically at Lady while she is wearing a muzzle. Thus, while Tramp believes that Lady should not have to wear a muzzle, he does not extend this belief onto other species. The speciesism in *Lady and the Tramp* is particularly evident from the film's depictions of working animals, which differ from the film's depictions of pets in significant ways. To illustrate, Trusty is a pet Bloodhound that lives in a large house near Lady. Like Lady, he clearly has a comfortable life as a pet, which is evident from his large house and high-quality dog collar. However, it is implied that Trusty, or at least his ancestors, were working dogs. On occasion, Trusty talks proudly about how his grandfather (Old Reliable) worked alongside detectives and solved many crimes. However, Jock confides in Lady that Trusty has lost his sense of smell. This implies that Trusty is now unable to work, which is why he is now a pet. This suggests that working animals that lose their abilities, specifically dogs, are given loving homes, which is a romanticization of the truth for many species of working animals. In reality, once working animals lose their abilities, they are often killed unceremoniously (Barnett 2006). However, as highlighted in Part I, dogs are the one exception to the unfair treatment working animals often experience. The film also suggests that Trusty wants to work, which is problematic because it suggests that working animals are subservient; in reality, working animals are not truly able to articulate what they want. WDAS has clearly depicted working dogs with much more respect than any other species of working animal. This is through detailed characterization, heavy anthropomorphism, and concern for any harms these animals experience. This is also notable in *The Fox and the Hound* (1981), for example. However, this is the opposite of how *Lady and the Tramp* depicts a different, but much more common, type of working animals: horses.

During the film's climax, Trusty chases the dog-catcher's horse-pulled cart. During this scene, Trusty intentionally frightens the non-anthropomorphised horses, which results in Trusty being seriously injured. However, the narrative encourages no sympathy for the non-anthropomorphised horses, which are barely shown after the accident. In contrast, the narrative encourages much sympathy for Trusty who is depicted as seriously injured by the crash. He lies in the street lifelessly as the other dogs watch solemnly. Jock (one of the other pet dogs) howls into the moonlight during this moment, suggesting that Trusty has died. In the original script for *Lady and the Tramp*, Trusty did die in this scene. However, one of the film's voice artists (Peggy Lee) was concerned about the effect that such a scene would have on young children, and so she asked Walt to change it, which he agreed to (Gavin 2015: 149, 480). Trusty is subsequently depicted in the film's final scene limping with a bandaged leg. This demonstrates again that WDAS has been cautious with their depictions of animal harm and death. However, the horses involved in the collision are never seen or mentioned again. Thus, their pain, injuries, and so forth are not reflected upon. This lack of detail, characterization, and anthropomorphism is how horses are portrayed throughout the film. For example, during the birth of Darling's baby, a horse is seen waiting outside in the rain. The horse is non-anthropomorphised and does not move, suggesting that it is an object, not an animal. These horses contrast significantly with the heavily-anthropomorphised and individually-characterized dog characters. The horses only exist to provide transport and realism. Thus, they are metaphorically objectified because they are not depicted expressing pain, emotions, and so forth, which the dog and cat characters are.

Many of the dog characters in *Lady and the Tramp* have had cameo appearances in later dog-centred WDAS films, including *Dalmatians* (1961) and *Oliver & Company* (1988). This highlights the lasting popularity of the dog characters compared to *Lady and the Tramp*'s working animals, which are never seen again. Additionally, the merchandise released during *Lady and the Tramp*'s release, and even today, focusses on the dog characters and occasionally the Siamese cats. For example, the official Disney merchandise shop today sells various toys and clothes relating to *Lady and the Tramp*, yet none feature the non-anthropomorphised horses (*Shop Disney* 2019e). Additionally, there is no evidence that the horses have ever been used to promote the film even though they are significant to the film's climax. This point, along with the film itself, demonstrates the speciesist attitudes WDAS often reflects and reinforces, especially towards pets and working animals. *Lady and the Tramp* implies that dogs deserve loving homes, free from harm, with kind, sensitive owners. This consideration is not given to the lower-order working-animals, such as horses. The horses are non-anthropomorphised, nameless, genderless, and without any distinguishing characteristics. There is no celebration of their species, or criticism of the routine harm or objectification that they can face. That is not to say that pets are offered a flattering portrayal as characters. The film includes both villainous and pro-social pets. Additionally, even the pro-social pets exhibit speciesist attitudes. However, this demonstrates that WDAS's pets are complex in characterization, which implies that these type of animals are capable of a much-wider range of emotions, and thus it is implied that they are sentient and perhaps have "personhood".

Conclusion

Pets and working animals have been depicted in WDAS films an almost equal amount of times. Further to this, dogs (WDAS's most common species of pet) are depicted in more WDAS films than any other species of animal. The second-most common species depicted in WDAS films are horses, which are WDAS's most common species of working animal. However, pets and working animals are treated very differently by humans, and this disparity has been accurately reflected in WDAS films. As the introduction of this chapter states, Peter Singer argued that some animals can be persons, and some cannot be. It is clear that a significant number of WDAS's pet characters could be considered persons, yet almost-all of their working animals could not be. In *Lady and the Tramp*, most of the dog characters are persons; they have homes, names, families, and so forth. Much of the main plot in *Lady and the Tramp* centres around Tramp's lack of home and family, i.e. his diminished state of personhood, which is happily resolved by the end of the film. However, the horses in *Lady and the Tramp* could not be considered persons as they do not possess these qualities, or rather, they have not been assigned those qualities by humans. This chapter's comparison between working animals and pets provides this book with the most convincing examples of speciesism in this text thus far. Pets and working animals are two groups of animals that have both lived alongside humans for thousands of years and still hold significant roles in human lives and culture. WDAS's pet characters are heavily anthropomorphised and assigned meaningful, individual, lives. In contrast, WDAS's working animals are often nameless, without individuality, and non-anthropomorphised. They exist in the background of WDAS films providing little more than context and realism. As this chapter demonstrated, they are depicted more often as objects (metaphorically) than as sentient animals. In contrast, while pets are less-anthropomorphised than many of WDAS's other animal characters, they are clearly given their own names and distinctive personalities. However, the positive portrayal that WDAS has given pets has not entirely benefitted pets in reality, which the "Disney effect" demonstrates.

This chapter has also evidenced that pets and working animals experience different types of harm in WDAS films. Additionally, WDAS's narratives encourage vastly different reactions to the harms that these two categories of animals experience. WDAS has implied that pets are undeserving of even minor harms, such as name-calling, unless they are villainous. If they are villainous, then mistreatment and even death is depicted as deserved. As with the other forms of animal harm studied in this book, there is also much romanticization, minimization, and attenuation of the common issues that pets face. For example, WDAS films imply that pet animals *choose* to be pets. Moreover, several films suggest that being a human's pet is the best possible life for an animal. In contrast, there is little romanticization of the harms that working animals experience, mainly because they are usually depicted as little more than objects (metaphorically). The existence of WDAS's working animals is necessary to the context of WDAS films, but not to the story. However, this un-sympathetic portrayal of working animals is perhaps reflective of how most humans view these animals in reality. Thus, WDAS's working animals exist purely to add realism, unless they are dogs. This is another example of how WDAS films are repeatedly speciesist.

5

Animal "Entertainers" in WDAS Films

A few days before the premiere of *A Dog's Purpose* (2017), there was an incident that would drastically change this film's legacy. On the 18th of January 2017, the entertainment website TMZ posted a minute-long clip of a dog being dragged and dipped into rushing water in order to film a scene for the movie. During the clip, an unidentified voice shouts: "Well, he ain't going to calm down until he goes in the water. Just got to throw him in" [sic] (Loughrey 2017). The off-stage voice then guffaws a few moments later as the dog (Hercules) is forced into the artificial rapids, seemingly against his will. The dog whines and attempts to break free of the trainer as he is lowered in. The video quickly went viral. This led to many organizations, such as PETA, to call for *A Dog's Purpose* to be boycotted (Polone 2017). Additionally, some of the film's own cast and crew spoke out in defence of the dog, rather than the film, during the controversy (Brucculieri 2017). As a result, the premiere of the film was cancelled, along with much of the movie's planned promotion (Shoard 2017). This dramatic instance highlights just how swiftly and strongly animal welfare organizations react to animals being mistreated for the purpose of producing entertainment. There are three main reasons why this incident became high-profile and led to instant action: the

R. R. Stanton, *The Disneyfication of Animals*, The Palgrave Macmillan Animal Ethics Series, https://doi.org/10.1007/978-3-030-49316-5_5

higher-order species involved, the visibility of the incident, and because it did not evoke the "collapse of compassion" effect.

This final chapter will explore how the use of animals in entertainment has been depicted in WDAS films. The use of animals for entertainment purposes is one of the most-debated and controversial areas of animal welfare. This is despite the fact that the entertainment industry uses far fewer animals than many other industries that use animals, such as factory farming. There are numerous ways that animals are used for entertainment; they are used in the film industry, circuses, zoos, oceanariums, horse racing, bullfighting, and so forth (*Animal Equality* 2019). This chapter will focus only on the six forms depicted in WDAS films: the film industry, stage performance, parades, street performance, circuses, and zoos.[1] Part I will examine why there is so much concern for animals in the entertainment industry and explore the problems with using animals as performers. Part II will document the number of times animal performance has been depicted in WDAS films. Then, Part III will explore the history of zoos and circuses. It will analyse how WDAS has depicted zoos and circuses and will include *Dumbo* (1941) as a case study. Finally, Part IV will study the use of animals in the American film industry. It will begin by examining the history of "animal actors" in the film industry, and then it will explore how WDAS has depicted animal actors. This section will use *Bolt* (2008) as a case study. This chapter will conclude by arguing that it is evidently becoming socially-unacceptable to use animals for entertainment purposes, which is evident from the portrayal of these industries in WDAS films.

Part I: Animals in Entertainment

As highlighted in Chap. 1, visible instances of animal harm significantly affect how people view industries that use animals. This is particularly evident from the film industry. As this chapter will demonstrate, entertainment companies need to be careful when training and working with animals as this can greatly shape their product's subsequent reception. For

[1] Horse riding was discussed in the previous chapter, so it will not be discussed further here.

example, the leaked footage from the filming of *A Dog's Purpose* negatively affected the planned release of this movie. *A Dog's Purpose* would have surely had its planned Hollywood premiere if the alleged animal mistreatment on-set had remained hidden from the public. By cancelling the film's premiere, the distributors seemed to be acknowledging that the actions in the leaked footage were unacceptable. Similarly, as Chap. 1 evidenced, one of the only reasons the farming industry is socially-acceptable is because its reality has been well-hidden behind romanticized images that minimize and distort the truth. This is the first reason why the use of animals for entertainment is such a sensitive area of animal welfare: since it is visible, the reality of it cannot be hidden, attenuated, or romanticized, as other ways of using animals have been.

The second reason why using animals for entertainment is controversial is because of the species involved. The species usually used in entertainment, such as big cats, tend to be higher-order species. Since entertainment is visible, animal performers need to be species that the public will want to view. Lower-order species within entertainment tend to be animated, neotenous, and anthropomorphised, such as Mickey Mouse and Roland Rat. In addition to the species, there are three factors of animal appearance that are also highly-favoured within animal performers: neoteny, colour, and size (Estren 2012: 9; MacClellan 2013: 57). The fact that physically-large, higher-order, neotenous, colourful animals are provided with higher standards of welfare is demonstrated by the fact that these species are usually socially-unacceptable to consume, hunt, and so forth (for example: Webb 2015). The only somewhat acceptable way to use these animals is in entertainment; however, as will be demonstrated in this chapter, this is gradually becoming unacceptable too.

The third reason why the use of animals in entertainment is such a sensitive issue is because the "collapse of compassion" effect usually does not occur. This is because animals in entertainment usually perform solo or in small groups. Moreover, many entertainment establishments, such as zoos, name their captive animals and give them personalized backstories, which further individualizes and anthropomorphises them (for example, see *Bristol Zoo Gardens* 2019). This personalization prohibits the "collapse of compassion" effect from occurring and thus makes the animals instinctively more engaging. The amount of time and money that has been spent trying to remove individual animal performers from captivity demonstrates this point. For example, the failed attempt at re-integrating Keiko (the whale that "starred" in *Free Willy*) back into the wild cost around 20 million dollars (Lusher 2003).[2] In contrast, animals used in industrialised farming contexts are almost never given the same consideration. Farm animals are purposefully grouped into uncountable nameless masses, which evokes the "collapse of compassion" response.

To summarize, the three main reasons why animal performance is subject to greater ethical scrutiny than other areas of animal harm and objectification is because it is visible, it involves higher-order species, and the animals are individualized (thereby negating the "collapse of compassion" effect). As evidenced in Chap. 2, these are also the reasons as to why hunting is no longer socially-acceptable. However, even though the use of animals in the entertainment industry attracts much concern from animal rights campaigners, it only affects a relatively small number of animals.[3] Despite this, many animal welfare campaigns are focussed in this area (for example: *PETA* 2019b, d, h, i). Moreover, the fact that the entertainment industry affects only a small number of animals does not mean that it shouldn't be challenged. Like other industries that use animals, the entertainment industry is harmful. There are six key reasons why using animals for entertainment is harmful: the training can involve harm, the animals are frequently forced to mimic human-like behaviours, the living conditions are often poor, the lives of the animals after

---

[2] Keiko was an orca that had been living in captivity since he was captured and removed from his mother in Iceland at the age of two. The release of *Free Willy* was followed by an outcry over comparisons between Keiko's own life and the story of Willy, which was presented as tragic and miserable in the film (Orlean 2002). For example, Keiko had been living in a small tank designed for dolphins and isolated from other whales for most of his life. This led to several campaigns to re-integrate Keiko back into the Icelandic waters that he had been taken from (Orlean 2002). The campaigns were successful, and Keiko's owners agreed to have him transferred back to Iceland. However, despite several attempts to integrate Keiko with natural whale pods, he lacked the social and survival skills to do so and kept returning to humans for food and comfort. After several failed integration attempts, Keiko was returned to captivity, and he died soon after (Orlean 2002). Most experts agree that Keiko had become too dependent on humans to have ever been successfully released into the wild (Brahic 2009).

[3] For example, there are only forty-eight zoos in the UK (*About Britain* 2019). In contrast, the UK has around 800 megafarms (Wasley et al. 2017).

performance, the risk animals pose to humans, and because it reinforces the anthropocentric idea that animals are human property.

One of the central issues with animal performers is the training involved. Since many animal performers are wild animals, they are difficult and time-consuming to train without the use of physical punishment and/or mutilation (*The Jane Goodall Institute Australia* 2018). For example, big cats are often declawed and usually have their teeth removed or filed down (*Born Free Foundation* 2016: 12). If an animal is mutilated or trained with the use of physical punishment, this occurs before the animal reaches a film set or circus big top; thus, it usually remains invisible to audiences. An infamous example of this is the 1989 case of Bobby Berosini. Berosini was a Las Vegas entertainer who was (unbeknownst to him) filmed backstage beating the orangutans used in his show (O'Connor 2016). During the trial spearheaded by PETA, Berosini's defence was that he was "correcting" the apes (Roderick 1990). This incident, and the high-profile trial it resulted in, raised public awareness of the physical mistreatment that many wild animals suffer during "training" and led to boycotts of similar shows (O'Connor 2016). This again highlights that the social acceptance of using animals for entertainment is dependent upon the treatment of any animals involved. When mistreatment is evident during training, as happened with Berosini's apes, the end product becomes infamous and is often blacklisted or boycotted.

The second problem is that animal performers are often required to perform human-like behaviours that are unnatural to them. For example, the *Moscow State Circus* trains their captive bears to walk on their hind legs while wearing human clothing and high heels (Cataldi 2002: 106). One reason why some humans enjoy this type of performance is because humans prefer animals with similar behaviour to their own (Batt 2009: 180–190). Higher-order species are viewed negatively when they engage in animalistic behaviour, such as mating "in public" (Beatson and Halloran 2010: 619–632). Thus, it is not enough to simply have higher-order animals as entertainers, they must also exhibit positive human behaviours and be trained to avoid their animalistic behaviours. To illustrate, the particularly animalistic behaviour of zoo animals, such as eating raw meat, often purposefully takes place "backstage" in zoos to avoid upsetting guests (Bettany and Belk 2011: 172–3). This explains why the most successful animal performers are mammals that have been trained to perform human-like behaviours, such as smiling and walking upright. However, this type of performance is often seen as undignified since it is unnatural to the animal. Yet others have claimed that embarrassment and self-respect are likely not felt by animals (Cataldi 2002: 115). This could be true of real animals but given that WDAS's animal characters are typically anthropomorphised, they are presented as being cognisant of their own dignity and embarrassment (as will be illustrated with *Dumbo* in Part III). Furthermore, these human-like skills, such as walking upright, are rarely useful to the animals themselves, except perhaps to relieve their own boredom (Stokes 2004: 152). Another issue with animals performing human-like behaviours is that it creates unrealistic expectations of that species. For example, non-human apes show their teeth to express discomfort, not happiness as humans do (Aldrich 2018: 5–21). Since animal performers are often trained to "smile" to mimic human behavioural norms, it is common to see apes "smiling" during performance (Aldrich 2018: 5–21). However, if an ape is trained to smile, it cannot be conclusively known if the ape is smiling because it is trained to or because it is anxious (and so is adhering to its species' behavioural norms). Humans rely upon behavioural cues to determine an animal's mental state. Therefore, if animals are trained to change these cues, their true state becomes impossible to decipher. Thus, it is difficult to ever assess a trained animal's specific welfare needs.

The third problem with animal entertainers is that they are often forced to perform and live in conditions far-removed from their natural habitats and lifestyles (*Born Free Foundation* 2016: 4). As a result, these animals often exhibit mental distress via behaviours such as repetitive swaying, incessant pacing, bar biting, and even self-harming (*Born Free Foundation* 2016: 4). In order to tame a wild animal, the animal is usually removed from its family group during infancy, sometimes when they are just a few days old. This is to force the animal to bond with humans and become familiar with their contact (*Born Free Foundation* 2016: 4). Because these animals are removed from their families while young, they do not learn the necessary survival skills that they would need if ever returned to the wild. This means that they cannot ever successfully be integrated back into their natural environment. This problem was demonstrated by the failed attempt at re-integrating Keiko, the whale that "starred" in *Free Willy* (1993).

The fourth problem with using animals for entertainment is what happens to them after their "careers" end. Once wild animals are too old for performance, they often spend the rest of their lives in zoos. Very few are ever released back into the wild or even into sanctuaries (*Born Free Foundation* 2016: 4, 13). Additionally, many animal performers, such as apes, can only be used as performers for a few years of their lives (*PETA* 2019h). This is because apes become rebellious and unpredictable in their teenage years. However, apes have a life expectancy of fifty to sixty years, meaning that many spend the rest of their lives in zoos and sanctuaries once they are too old for performance (Pinto 2004). Michael Jackson's pet chimpanzee, Bubbles, is one example of this problem. Bubbles was rescued by Jackson as an infant and became well-known as Jackson's pet in the eighties (Hadley 2009: 41). Bubbles would often wear human clothes and "perform" to humans. However, once Bubbles matured, he became aggressive, unpredictable, and badly-behaved. As a result, Bubbles was put into an animal sanctuary where he still lives today. Bubbles currently lives at the *Center for Great Apes* in Florida, a sanctuary for many of the great apes that used to work in the entertainment industry (Hadley 2009: 41).

The fifth issue is that animal performers pose significant dangers to humans (*Born Free Foundation* 2016: 6). For example, in 2003, the entertainer Roy Horn was viciously attacked and dragged off-stage by one of his tigers during a live magic performance (Peterson 2007: 33). The attack left Horn paralysed and abruptly ended his Las Vegas show, which had been one of the most successful shows in Vegas history (Preschel 2005). Additionally, there is a risk of disease transmission (zoonotic diseases) between animals and humans, which can be fatal for both parties (*Born Free Foundation* 2016: 6). This suggests that interaction between humans and wild animals needs to be appropriately distanced.

The sixth problem with using animals as entertainers is that it implies that animals are human property. In 1929, it was rumoured that Rin Tin Tin, an internationally-famous German Shepherd that had "starred" in more than twenty feature films, received the most nominations for "Best Actor" during the Academy Awards "Oscars" ballot (Brooks 2012). More recently, Uggie, the Jack Russell Terrier that starred in *The Artist* (2011), inspired several campaigns that aimed to award him an Oscar or BAFTA for his film performance (Hawkes 2016). However, neither animal actor received an award or were even formally nominated. This highlights two points: the public's love and respect for animal actors, but also the discrimination that these "actors" face. Even though animal actors are named "actors" and are protected by SAG,[4] they are not treated the same as human actors are. In fact, the Academy Awards' guidelines even specify that only actors and actresses (i.e. humans) are eligible for these awards, which is why Rin Tin Tin and Uggie were never awarded Oscars for their performances (Diamond 2017). The fact that these animals are denied awards suggests that they are seen as objects, rather than actors.

These six points demonstrate the central issues with using animals for performance. On the basis of these issues, animal welfare groups, such as PETA, have been campaigning for films, circuses, and so forth, to entirely stop using real animals (for example: *PETA* 2019d, o). These campaigns have so far been relatively successful. For example, in 2012, Disney responded to the growing backlash against the use of ape actors by announcing that they would no longer be using apes or large primates in any of their live-action films (Aldrich 2018: 5–21). This is one indication that the use of animals in entertainment is becoming socially-unacceptable. Indeed, as Parts III and IV of this chapter will demonstrate, WDAS films have mostly reflected this attitude.

Part II: Data

Below are all of the depictions of animal actors, circuses, zoos, and so forth in the fifty-six WDAS films included in this study.[5] This data only includes instances of animals performing for humans. For example, the stage performance in *The Great Mouse Detective* (1986) is not being included as it involves mice performing for other mice.

---

[4] SAG is the Screen Actors' Guild, an American labour union for film performers. SAG will be further discussed in Part IV of this chapter.

[5] "Willie the Whale Who Wanted to Sing at the Met" from *Make Mine Music* (1946) is not being included here since Willie's performance takes place during a dream sequence.

- *Dumbo* (1941): Zoos and circuses
- *Fun and Fancy Free* (1947): Circuses
- *Lady and the Tramp* (1955): Zoos
- *The Rescuers* (1977): Zoos
- *Aladdin* (1992): Zoos and a parade
- *Fantasia 2000* (1999): Street performance
- *Meet the Robinsons* (2007): Stage performance
- *Bolt* (2008): Animal actors in the film industry

From this data, it is evident that zoos have been depicted in four films, circuses have been depicted in two films, and the use of animals in film, animals on stage, animals in parades, and animal street performance have been depicted in one film each. Therefore, it is apparent from this data that WDAS has not often depicted the use of animals in entertainment. This is in stark contrast to how often they have depicted other ways that humans use animals, even socially-unacceptable ones such as hunting, as the previous four chapters of this book show. This may be because this area is controversial and upsetting to many, which has been the case for all of WDAS's history (1937–present). As highlighted in Chap. 1, WDAS has obscured the harsh reality of modern farming behind unrealistic, romanticized images. However, as evidenced in Part I of this chapter, it is difficult to romanticize animal performance because it is visible. Indeed, this may be why the most controversial forms of entertainment that use animals, such as bull fighting,[6] dog fighting, and so forth, have never been depicted by WDAS. Similarly, as highlighted in Chap. 1, socially-acceptable forms of farming, such as dairy farming, are often depicted in WDAS films, yet socially-unacceptable farming practices, such as the production of veal and foie gras, have never been. As highlighted in Part I of this chapter, the use of animals in film, circuses, zoos, and so forth is becoming socially-unacceptable, which perhaps indicates that they are unlikely to be depicted frequently by WDAS in the near future. This

[6] In *The Three Caballeros* (1945), there is a scene in which Donald Duck pretends to be a bull and wears a mechanical bull costume. During this scene, Jose Carioca (a parrot) pretends to be the bull fighter and holds up a red flag for Donald to run towards. This is not being included here as it is mocking bull fighting rather than depicting it. The "bull" is Donald Duck in a paper costume; thus, it is not a real bull.

chapter will now discuss the most common forms of animal entertainment that have been depicted by WDAS: circuses and zoos.

Part III: Circuses, Zoos, and *Dumbo* (1941)

The opposition towards using animals for entertainment is not a recent phenomenon: it is evident in ancient history. For example, the ancient Roman philosopher Cicero noted after a visit to the notoriously-violent games that the audience felt compassion for the elephants involved (Stevens and McAlister 2007: 95).[7] Additionally, some of the first modern animal welfare laws in the UK concerned animals in entertainment. For example, in 1835 all forms of animal baiting were banned in Britain (Stevens and McAlister 2007: 96). Today, there appears to be increasing opposition to the use of animals for entertainment. This is particularly evident from social media and animal rights activism (Wilson 2017: 363). Because of this, many circuses, zoos, and similar environments have adopted a welfare-focussed image or, in some cases, stopped using animals altogether.

Modern public zoos became widespread after the age of enlightenment when people began to study animals for scientific purposes (*National Geographic* 2019). These zoos grew alongside the rise in cities, offering green places away from noise and pollution (Vandersommers 2017). Over time, zoo enclosures have changed from simple concrete living spaces to ones that closely resemble the natural habitat of the species kept (Gray 2014: 43–4). Even though there was opposition towards keeping animals captive in ancient history, it was not until the end of the nineteenth century that zoos became welfare-focussed (Vandersommers 2017). For example, it was not until 1907 that a zoo without cages opened (Phillips 2015). This cageless zoo design, which separated animals from the public with moats, was influential and inspired the design of the modern welfare-focussed zoos that are common today (Phillips 2015). In 2017, there were around 10,000 zoos worldwide, which were

[7] The Roman games were barbaric spectacles that killed humans and animals in bizarre and cruel ways for the purpose of entertainment (Stevens and McAlister 2007: 95).

host to around 675 million guests annually (Vandersommers 2017). Thus, zoos are clearly still both common and popular attractions, despite their modern controversies.

There are several arguments often made against modern zoos. First, wild animals, such as lions and chimpanzees, react badly to life in a zoo (Pierce and Bekoff 2018: 45). There are a small number of species, such as snails,[8] that appear to thrive in zoos; however, the species that thrive tend to be of little interest to the public (Pierce and Bekoff 2018: 45–6). Therefore, while zoos can adequately house some species, it is mainly the ones that do not benefit which are kept. Second, animals bred in captivity are unlikely to ever be re-introduced back into the wild (Stoddart 2004: 26–7). In fact, most animals in zoos today were born there rather than taken from the wild (Phillips 2015). Third, as with other forms of animal entertainment, zoos only tend to hold and conserve animals that the public will want to view, such as lions, elephants, and baby animals (Gray 2014: 48). Zoo animals that are purposefully euthanized tend to be killed as they enter adulthood as this is when they become of less interest to the public (Gray 2014: 52–3). For example, in 2014, *Copenhagen Zoo* legally euthanized a healthy two-year old giraffe named Marius. The zoo defended this decision by claiming that Marius's genetic material was redundant (Gunasekera 2018: 93). In light of these three common criticisms, many zoos have adopted a welfare-focussed image. Within this image, there are several arguments often raised in support of zoos. First, it is argued that zoos house species that are extinct in wild. These are usually species that would likely face extinction if released; thus, zoos provide their only chance of survival. Second, it is often argued that modern zoos are educational and raise awareness of conservation issues (Stoddart 2004: 26–7). Third, it is said that circuses and zoos offer animals better lives than in the wild since they provide medical attention, easy access to food, and so forth (Nijland et al. 2013: 529). Thus, it has been argued that if a zoo mimics an animal's biological and social needs, then the animal's rights are not violated (Gunasekera 2018: 95–6). However, recent research has claimed that most zoos are "horrific" places, with just 3%

[8] Since snails are small in size and have a limited home range, zoo environments do not seem to affect them negatively (Pierce and Bekoff 2018: 46).

meeting the ethical standards set (Pierce and Bekoff 2018: 45; Gray 2017: 208).[9] This suggests that most zoos do not meaningfully replicate the environment that captive animals need and are thus, for the most part, harmful.

A 2015 survey that found that 69% of Americans were concerned about animals in the circus. This was higher than the concern for other industries that use animals in far higher numbers, such as research and food (Yuhas 2015). Circuses are commonly seen as less-ethical than zoos and the film industry even though the animals involved often overlap (*Born Free Foundation* 2016: 3). This is likely because of the "performance" involved, which, as evidenced in Part I, usually involves animals mimicking human behaviours that are unnatural to them (Cataldi 2002: 104–6). Additionally, and also unlike zoos, circuses travel. Some circuses travel for up to fifty weeks each year, which is believed to be very uncomfortable for the animals involved (Gray 2014: 41). Like zoos, circuses are also responding to the growing backlash against animal performance by finding more ethical alternatives. For example, the *Cirque du Soleil* is probably the most financially-successful modern circus, and it uses no animals at all (*One Green Planet* 2019). Additionally, Ringling Brothers and Barnum & Bailey Circus, a circus that was infamous for its use of live animals, permanently closed in 2017 (Davis 2017: 346).[10]

During the nineteenth century in America, there were many dramatic instances that occurred in touring menageries and circuses, such as escaped wild animals and collapsing tents (Coleman 2015: 606–7). These chaotic instances were written up as spectacular stories, creating exciting publicity for these forms of entertainment (Coleman 2015: 606–7). Thus, audiences began to expect thrilling incidents at these places, which arguably further pushed the boundaries of danger within animal performance. This danger is still drawn upon in advertisements for zoos and

[9] Jenny Gray, chief executive officer of Zoos Victoria, claims that just 3% of zoos are striving to meet ethical standards in her 2017 text *The Challenges of Compassionate Conservation* (Pierce and Bekoff 2018: 45; Gray 2017: 208).

[10] Ringling Brothers and Barnum & Bailey Circus was created by P. T. Barnum in the nineteenth century. In 2016, a year before their closure, they agreed to stop using elephants, but they continued to use tigers, lions, and other wild animals. The circus's 2017 closure was blamed on high operating costs and decreased attendance (*The Guardian* 2017).

circuses. For example, zoos often describe their animals as being wild and dangerous, even though the animals are caged, and therefore pose little danger to the public (Wilson 2017: 350). Additionally, dramatic incidents are often used in narratives centred around zoos and circuses, as can be seen in *Dumbo* (1941) and *We Bought a Zoo* (2011), for example. However, when an animal does escape or behave in a dangerous manner, zoos and circuses usually respond by putting the welfare of the animal second to the customer. For example, in 1994, Tyke (an elephant) killed her trainer, seriously harmed her groomer, escaped from the circus, and then rampaged through the streets of Honolulu (Hawaii). Tyke was killed soon after by being shot 87 times by the police (Cave 2017). This dramatic incident attracted much publicity worldwide.

As highlighted in Part II, WDAS has seldom depicted zoos and circuses, even though they have often depicted the species that can commonly be seen in these locations, such as lions. WDAS's first portrayal of zoos and circuses was in one of their earliest films, *Dumbo* (1941). *Dumbo* was adapted from *Dumbo, the Flying Elephant*, an illustrated "Roll-a-Book", by Helen Aberson and Harold Pearl (Langer 1990: 310).[11] It is likely that the book was likely inspired by one of P. T. Barnum's notable elephants, Jumbo, who was believed to have been the most successful circus attraction in American history (Brooke 2001). For example, Jumbo was directly credited with helping Barnum's show gross $336,000 in his first six weeks (Brooke 2001). The original *Dumbo* roll-a-book by Aberson and Pearl contained just a few lines of text and eight pictures. Perhaps because of its unusual format, no copies of the original roll-a-book are known to exist (Barrier 2011). However, it is believed that the story was similar to WDAS's later adaptation (Barrier 2011). *Dumbo* was produced at the same time *as Bambi*, but it is notable for having much lower-quality animation. Despite this, *Dumbo* was WDAS's most profitable film of the forties (Barrier 2011).[12] Even though the animation of *Dumbo*

[11] A "roll-a-book" is a picture book built into a box that the reader twists to get to the next slide (Barrier 2011).

[12] The main purpose of *Dumbo* was to generate much-needed revenue for the financially-troubled WDAS studios. This was why the animation quality on *Dumbo* is much lower than on other WDAS works of the time. WDAS was financially-troubled because they had invested much of their money into both *Fantasia* and *Bambi* (Langer 1990: 310). Unlike its much more expensive prede-

was of a much lower-quality than on *Bambi*, some of the production techniques were similar. For example, there was a small zoo in the animation studio so that the artists could draw directly from live animals, including elephants (Pallant 2011: 47).

As highlighted earlier in this chapter, objections towards animals in entertainment are notable throughout history. Thus, even though *Dumbo* was released in 1941, the use of animals for entertainment was a topical issue at this time. *Dumbo* highlights some of the common problems with using animals in circuses/ zoos, yet, like other WDAS films about industries that use animals, such as *Dalmatians*, it avoids being too critical or gruesome. The beginning of *Dumbo* presents a balanced view of circus/ zoo life in which the lives of captive animals are romanticized, yet mistreatment is also suggested. For example, a still image in the film's opening credits depicts a circus ringmaster with a whip stalking a tiger. However, in the actual film, no animals are whipped at all. These still images are accompanied by the sound of an upbeat brass band, which suggests excitement rather than a harmful situation. This suggestion of mistreatment is even further contrasted during the film's opening, which romanticizes zoos, circuses, and parenthood. In the film's first scene, anthropomorphised storks are seen delivering blanket-wrapped newborn offspring to the various captive zoo/circus animals, much to the animals' delight. During this scene, the cages the animals are kept in are quite small, yet the animals themselves appear to be comfortable and happy. For example, some are smiling, and some are sleeping peacefully. There is no bar baiting or other unnatural behaviours that real captive animals are evidenced to suffer from. This scene suggests that wild animals are comfortable and happy in captivity, even when housed in small confined spaces unreflective of their natural habitat. Furthermore, in contrast to the film's opening image, the tigers in *Dumbo* are not chased with whips by ringmasters. Instead, they appear to live free from physical harm in nuclear family units. Throughout the film, the animals remain with their young and are not separated, with the notable exception of

---

cessor *Fantasia*, *Dumbo* was released to positive reviews; however, its strong publicity was somewhat cut short by the unexpected attack on Pearl Harbour that occurred a few weeks after its release (*The Walt Disney Family Museum* 2011).

Mrs. Jumbo and Dumbo.[13] As evidenced in Part I, circus animals are usually separated from their families when young to prepare them for a lifetime of human contact. Therefore, this portrayal of zoos is not reflective of how captive animals are usually treated in reality. This inaccuracy matters because it misrepresents the harsh lives that many captive animals experience. As the previous chapter demonstrated with the "Disney effect", many people develop their knowledge of animals from cultural representations such as WDAS films. Therefore, if WDAS films are portraying zoos/circuses as locations in which captive animals stay with their families for life, these false ideas could mis-educate viewers on the harsh reality of these locations. It is not Disney's responsibility to educate people; however, Disney should be cautious of the fact that their depictions of animals may be the only exposure to some species that many people have.

The next morning, the captive animals and their new offspring willingly board a specially-built circus train to travel to their next city. Different species are seen mixing harmoniously during this moment. For example, the camels board and share a cart with the zebras, which both species appear to be comfortable with. This is another romanticization of natural animal behaviour. In reality, camels and zebras are unlikely to socialize in the wild because of their disparate native locations. However, the film does not present this as a problem as both species appear happy with their shared travelling conditions. Upon arrival at their new circus location, the animals subserviently help the human circus workers to set up the big top. Each species uses their distinguishing characteristics to facilitate the process. For example, the camels use their humps to carry poles. This scene suggests that the captive animals are willing participants within the circus, rather than being forced to work and perform. Throughout this scene, the animals are not caged, chained, or restricted in any way. They move around freely with the humans, and none attempt to escape. Thus, the animals do not only perform when onstage (by enacting trained behaviours): they are part of the operation *in toto*. The human circus workers work alongside the animals in this scene. This suggests

[13] As revealed early in the film, Dumbo's name is actually Jumbo Jr. However, given that he is almost-always referred to as "Dumbo", that is the name that will be used here for clarity.

that both humans and other animals are equal employees in the circus, rather than the humans dominating or controlling the animals. This scene also implies that the cages the animals were in in the first scene were not necessary, which makes the them seem even less-harmful. Thus, the cages in *Dumbo* are depicted as both comfortable and unnecessary, which, as the evidence presented earlier suggests, is the opposite of reality.

During the circus's opening parade the next day, the wild animals are paraded through their new location, with some of the animals being transported in moving cages. During this scene, a seemingly angry gorilla accidently breaks the bars on its cage while growling at the crowds. The gorilla is shocked by this breakage and dutifully replaces the bar. This implies both that the gorilla is happy to be caged, and also that it is willingly and knowingly performing. The cage appears to be a part of the gorilla's performance, rather than a harmful restriction of the gorilla's freedom. The gorilla's shocked reaction suggests that it is knowingly performing rather than acting naturally. This implies that the gorilla's wildness is just an act, and that its natural state is caged domestication. Additionally, this scene suggests that the anger captive animals exhibit is part of their performance, rather than because of their unnatural living conditions. Furthermore, this scene implies that the animals in *Dumbo* are knowingly part of an industry that uses animals, and they are happy to work in it, rather than restricted or enslaved by it. This was also how animals in the dairy industry were depicted in *Home on the Range,* as demonstrated in Chap. 1.

Further to this, and also similar to *Range*, the main storyline of *Dumbo* suggests that animals are responsible for their own misfortune. After the circus parade, Mrs. Jumbo is forcibly separated from Dumbo after attacking a zoo guest that mocks Dumbo's big ears. This attack leads to a stampede in the tent, and it takes at least twenty men to restrain Mrs. Jumbo. As highlighted earlier, chaotic scenes like this are common in circus/zoo narratives and are occasionally evident in reality. However, this moment is problematic because it partly justifies the later punishment of Mrs. Jumbo. Because of her aggression towards humans, Mrs. Jumbo is locked in an isolated cage with her movements restricted by a ball and chain. A sign on her small dark cage reads "MAD ELEPHANT". However, the narrative implies that Mrs. Jumbo is partly at-fault for her imprisonment.

Because of the stampede she caused prior to her imprisonment, the film depicts violence towards humans before it displays any mistreatment towards animals. As highlighted in Chap. 2, when animals are initiators of violence (towards humans or animals), the narrative subsequently encourages less sympathy towards them. In reality, zoo/circus animals are frequently separated from their offspring. However, in *Dumbo*, it is implied that this separation only occurs when the mother misbehaves; if Mrs. Jumbo had not acted aggressively, she would surely not have been separated from her baby. Thus, *Dumbo* misleads viewers on the real reasons why captive animals are separated from their infants; it blames this regular practice on the actions of animals rather than the industries themselves. Further to this, the other elephants (except Dumbo) blame Mrs. Jumbo's solitary confinement on Dumbo rather than the captive circus/zoo environment. The elephants explicitly state this opinion when gossiping about Mrs. Jumbo within earshot of Dumbo:

Prissy:	Well, l-I must say, l-I don't blame her for anything.
Catty:	You're absolutely right. It's all the fault of that little F-R-E-A-K.
Off-screen elephant:	Yes, him with those ears that only a mother could love.

This narrative distracts from underlying problems inherent to the circus environment, which deflects the misfortune and subsequent unhappiness that captive animals can experience onto the animals themselves. The other elephants imply that Mrs. Jumbo should not have attacked the guests to defend Dumbo. At no point do they criticize the ignorant actions of the zoo guest that mocked Dumbo, who, from an animal welfare perspective, was the one at fault in the situation.

After his mother is caged, Dumbo is made to perform an "elephant pyramid" with the other elephants. During this act, the elephants climb on top of each other to create a pyramid shape. Dumbo is supposed to stand on the top of the other elephants with a flag; however, as he approaches the "pyramid", he trips on his big ears and falls into it instead. This leads the "pyramid" to collapse, resulting in chaos for the circus and much pain for the other elephants. As with the imprisonment of Mrs. Jumbo, this scene blames Dumbo for the chaos, rather than the environment itself. If these wild animals were living in their natural habitats, it is unlikely that they would be making "elephant pyramids" and thus would not have been harmed. As highlighted in Part I, the tricks learned by captive animals are rarely useful to the animals themselves. Thus, the circus is at fault here. However, in *Dumbo* the animals are the ones blamed, and indeed they blame each other for the problems they experience. Additionally, given Dumbo's young age, naivety, and oversized ears (which make him clumsy), it seems particularly harmful for him to be a part of a circus act such as this one. The way that the elephants speak to each other during the "elephant pyramid" scene is humorous, which further distracts from the harms of the scene. For example, one says: "Gaining a little weight, aren't you honey?" as another elephant climbs on top of her. By implying that one of the elephants has gained weight, the text subtly suggests that these elephants are not underfed, and thus their basic needs are being sufficiently met by the circus environment. Additionally, this question implies that the amount of food the elephants eat is at their own discretion. This implies that the elephants have the freedom to exercise autonomy, and also that the circus is offering plenty of food (negating any implication that the animals might be neglected). After their doomed "elephant pyramid" ends in disaster, the elephants are comically bandaged up in a cartoonish fashion. For example, one of them has her skinny tail in a sling. Again, this comedy removes the anxiety that viewers may hold over the harms that have come to the animals. It also further suggests that the elephants are well cared-for off-stage, perhaps overly so, given the excessive amount of bandages they wear.

Because of the elephant pyramid collapse, Dumbo is demoted to a clown, which the other elephants find shameful. This leads to Dumbo being ostracised from the herd. The other elephants put their trunks together to promise that they will no longer associate with Dumbo because of his clown status. This demonstrates that the other elephants take great pride in their circus act and are willing performers. They see being human (i.e. a clown) as more shameful than having to perform an "elephant pyramid". They did not ostracise Dumbo when he was part of the "elephant pyramid", only when he became a clown and thus performed alongside humans rather than other elephants. Thus, these circus animals are presented as having pride in their exclusively-animal performance. This suggests that circus animals do have feelings, such as pride, but that their feelings are in support of the circus rather than their own interests, such as their potential life in the wild. Therefore, the film appears to support the use of animals in the circus, as long as the animals involved are content with their situation, which by the end of the film, all of the animals are.

Dumbo is the least anthropomorphised of any of WDAS's animal protagonists. This is mainly because he (and his mother) do not speak, yet all of the other elephants and some of the other animal characters do. Dumbo and his mother face the worst treatment in the circus; however, because they do not speak, their unhappiness is implied (such as through crying) rather than stated. In other WDAS films about the ethics of using animals, harm is more evident because of the voice the characters have. For example, in *Bambi* and *Brother Bear*, the animals explicitly state their fear of hunters verbally. In *Dumbo*, the animals that are happy with their lives in the circus, such as the rest of the elephant herd and Timothy Q. Mouse (Dumbo's sidekick), do speak. Furthermore, as the previous paragraphs highlight, it is obvious from their conversations that they are not ashamed of, or unhappy with, their circus lives. For example, it is Timothy Q. Mouse who coaches Dumbo as a performer and makes him the star of the circus. If Dumbo and his mother did speak, they would surely speak negatively about the circus and perhaps express a desire to leave. Yet by not speaking, there is less blame applied to the circus. Thus, the two characters who would complain about the circus environment literally cannot voice their criticisms.

Similar to *Bambi*, the humans in *Dumbo* are less-developed than the animal characters. They are nameless and often appear as shadows. This lack of characterization de-humanizes these characters and encourages the audience to engage less with them. This is because nameless groups of characters evoke less compassion than individuals (Borkfelt 2011: 116–125). This is similar to the characterization of the grouped, faceless, nameless, human villains in *Bambi* (which was being produced at the same time). After Dumbo is demoted to a clown and forced to jump a large distance from a diving board, the human clowns excitedly decide to make his jump even higher, and thus even more dangerous, in order to further impress the crowd. When one human clown suggests that this stunt may harm Dumbo, another declares that "Elephants ain't got no feelings", and then another quickly adds: "They're made o' rubber" [sic]. Thus, these clowns are ignorant to the sentience and pain of the animals they are using. Their only interest in Dumbo is with his potential as a performer. Thus, most of them view circus animals as objects rather than sentient beings. However, the film makes it clear that these animals do have feelings, can feel pain, and so forth. This is particularly evident from the emotional mother-son relationship between Dumbo and his mother. This ignorance, along with the clowns' lack of character, makes the clowns villainous. However, as quoted above, one of the clowns believes that elephants are made of rubber; therefore, they do not understand that their actions are harmful. This stops their villainy from being malicious or repellent. This contrasts with the villains in *Bambi*, for example, who do seem to know that their actions are harmful. Thus, the clowns are intriguing villains, like Cruella. As highlighted earlier, *Dumbo* was much more successful than *Bambi*, which was released soon after. The villains in *Bambi* are known for being terrifying (i.e. repellent) as Chap. 2 demonstrated. They even feature at 20th place on the AFI's list of greatest villains alongside the likes of Hannibal Lector and Norman Bates (*American Film Institute* 2019). In contrast, the clowns in *Dumbo*, whilst ignorant, are not terrifying. This could have contributed to the unexpected success of *Dumbo* over *Bambi*. As Chap. 3 demonstrated, WDAS's intriguing villains, such as Cruella, have evidently been far more popular with audiences than their repellent ones. For example, Cruella has been revived many times and still features in much Disney merchandise today. In contrast, the human villains from *Bambi* are not remembered fondly. There is no known merchandise that features them, nor have they been featured in subsequent Disney media, which is in stark contrast to engaging characters like Cruella. Thus, even though the clowns are intriguing, their lack of characterization seems to have made them forgettable.

The film ends with Dumbo becoming the "star" of the circus, but only after he learns to use his big ears to his advantage as a performer. Additionally, Mrs. Jumbo is released from her "MAD ELEPHANT" cage after Dumbo becomes a star. She is last depicted riding comfortably in

Dumbo's luxurious train carriage as he happily flies above her. Thus, Dumbo's life in the circus improves because his circus skills improve. If he had continued to perform badly, it is unlikely that he would have become a "star" and given many luxuries. Therefore, in *Dumbo*, both the happiness and unhappiness of captive animals is based upon their own actions and choices. In reality, the lives captive animals live are dictated entirely by humans. Yet *Dumbo* implies that captive animals have a choice in their future, which in reality, they do not. Thus, *Dumbo* ends by depicting circuses as happy, comfortable, locations for animals, as long as they behave themselves and learn to perform well. This is not to say that *Dumbo* entirely romanticizes the circus/zoo environment as there is some acknowledgement of how these locations can potentially harm animals. For example, the depiction of circus guests as mindless and ignorant seems to reference that these places do not always encourage visitors to respect the animals. However, the six main problems experienced by animal performers, as detailed in Part I, are either ignored, minimized, or romanticized in *Dumbo*. For example, whilst captive animals are depicted living in small, caged, spaces, un-reflective of their natural habitat, they are portrayed as being happy with this situation. Moreover, these cages are escapable and sometimes the animals are free to roam outside of them. Furthermore, it is notable that whenever Dumbo performs a new trick to a large crowd, he is performing that trick for the first time. Thus, the text has removed one of the most-common problems with using animals in entertainment: training. Additionally, the film also does not depict what happens to the animals once they can no longer perform. Mrs. Jumbo's imprisonment is portrayed as her own fault, rather than routine practice for older animals. The only animals that are depicted as unhappy with their lives are Dumbo and his mother, which is portrayed as their own fault and is fully resolved by the end of the film. Throughout the entire narrative, all of the other captive animals are happy to live in cages and proud to perform dangerous tricks in the big top. In fact, the circus animals even encourage each other to do so. Thus, despite some acknowledgement of the harms that circus/ zoo animals can experience, the portrayal of circuses/zoos in *Dumbo* could only be considered as a favourable depiction of these locations.

Six years after *Dumbo*, WDAS released *Fun and Fancy Free*. This film contained the short "Bongo", which also centres around the lives of circus animals.[14] Like Dumbo, Bongo is the star of the circus, and he is happy to perform dangerous stunts, such as jumping from great heights. However, after his performance, the narrator reveals that Bongo the bear is treated quite badly by insensitive circus workers (who, as in *Dumbo*, are also faceless and nameless). The narrator announces that Bongo is "tossed around like an old shoe" after each circus performance. However, this mistreatment is not explicitly depicted. Bongo is then shown in a cage, but one that has several luxuries, such as a bed and dressing table. Thus, even though the film states that Bongo is being mistreated, his mistreatment is still downplayed. Real circus animals that are neglected are unlikely to have spacious bedrooms with furniture, nor any chance of escape. It is clear that Bongo dreams of a life in his natural habitat. These thoughts encourage him to escape, which he does with relative ease. However, Bongo initially struggles to adapt to life in the wild since he is unable to perform natural animal behaviours, such as climbing trees and fishing by hand. Thus, it is implied that his earlier life in the circus was easier than his chosen life in his natural habitat. Given that *Bongo* was intended as a sequel to *Dumbo*, it is unsurprising that they have many similarities. Like Dumbo, Bongo is mute, is unhappy with his initial situation, and is bullied by other animals. Additionally, as in *Dumbo*, Bongo's difficulties are fully-resolved by the end of the text. The problem with *Bongo* is similar to those in *Dumbo* in that the challenges the circus animals face do not come entirely from the circus. Even though it is explicitly stated that Bongo is mistreated by the circus, the actual harm Bongo experiences on-screen is from wild bears, not human circus workers. For example, Bongo almost dies in the wild after getting into a fight with a wild bear. Thus, the film presents the wild as a more dangerous place for animals, which is problematic because it suggests

[14] This was the first half of *Fun and Fancy Free* (1947), one of WDAS's "Wartime Era" package films. *Bongo* was originally intended to be a feature-length sequel to *Dumbo*. However, the script was finalized one day after the attack on Pearl Harbour; therefore, on the very same day, the Disney studios became occupied by the U.S. military. During this time, the studio was commissioned to make propaganda films, meaning that *Bongo* and a few other planned films were shelved. Once back in production, it was decided that the animation of *Bongo* and *Mickey and the Beanstalk* was not good enough to be a feature film, so they were paired together to create *Fun and Fancy Free* (*AFI: American Film Institute* 1999: 838).

that circuses are a safer option for wild animals. This is similar to *Home on the Range*, in which a dairy farm is depicted as a safer location than the wild for farm animals. The problems for both Bongo and Dumbo stem from the fact that they are circus animals; however, both texts blame the animals themselves for their own misfortune.

In March 2019, Walt Disney Studios released their live-action remake of 1941's *Dumbo*. Upon hearing of the plans for the film, PETA urged the director (Tim Burton) to change the original ending and allow Dumbo and his mother to escape the circus at the film's end (Sanchez 2018). The original ending of WDAS's 1941 *Dumbo* implies that both Dumbo and his mother are happy to continue living and performing in the circus, despite their earlier mistreatment. This ending is problematic from an animal welfare perspective for the reasons highlighted here and in Part I. It seems that Disney listened to the concerns from animal rights' groups; the ending of 2019's *Dumbo* depicts Dumbo and his mother leaving the circus and travelling to India to join a wild elephant herd. Moreover, the circus they escape from vows to never use captive animals again. This hopeful, optimistic, ending is romantic and does not reflect the real lives most circus animals have after retirement. However, it does highlight that Disney is adapting their texts to align with the social-acceptance of using animals for performance. Disney's revised ending also highlights just how much attitudes towards keeping animals captive have changed in just a few decades.

Part IV: Animal Actors and *Bolt* (2008)[15]

Animals have been involved in the film industry since it began (Burt 2002: 87). They often open scenes, or even introduce whole films, as illustrated by MGM's famous roaring lion logo (Burt 2002: 19). As this chapter has already demonstrated, there have been many campaigns against the use of animals in entertainment (Burt 2002: 165–7). When there is visible evidence that animals were harmed during filmmaking, there is usually backlash towards the film. The swift, passionate backlash

[15] Some of this section is due to be published elsewhere. It is currently under peer review.

against *A Dog's Purpose* demonstrates this point. As a result of this sensitivity, many film companies often boast that their animal actors are treated just as well as their human performers are. It has even been argued that the film industry provides animals with a "universal sanctuary" since animal actors are often protected from the normalized mistreatment and neglect that their species routinely face in other industries (Schnug 2011: 21). The amount of concern consumers exhibit towards animal actors is perhaps best evidenced by the support and respect given to the American Humane Association (hereafter: AHA), an organization focussed on the welfare of animal actors.

The AHA was founded in 1877 to advocate on behalf of animals and children. Their first animal-focussed aim was to improve the treatment of farm animals during livestock transportation (*American Humane* 2019d). Today, the AHA is a non-profit organization that mainly monitors the use of animals on American film sets (*American Humane* 2019f). Their website proudly claims that they support the welfare of all species of animal actors, from ants to zebras (*American Humane* 2019f). Before the AHA began monitoring animals in the film industry, animals were commonly mistreated on film sets (Rees 2017: 355). The AHA first started investigating animal harm within the film industry in the 1920s after seeing how many horses were injured and killed during the production of "wild west" films. For example, during the production of *Jesse James* (1939), a blindfolded horse died after being intentionally ridden over a seventy-foot drop into a river (*American Humane* 2019d). After this particular incident, there was increased public concern towards the use of animals in the film industry (Baum 2013a). This subsequently helped the AHA to gain the authority to monitor film sets (*American Humane* 2019d). Since 1980, the Screen Actors Guild (hereafter: SAG)[16] has given the AHA the sole authority of overseeing animal welfare in Hollywood films (*American Humane* 2019d). Today, the AHA claims to be an

[16] SAG (also sometimes known as SAG-AFTRA) is an American labor union that represents a large number of professional media performers, such as film actors (*SAG-AFTRA* 2018). All SAG films, television shows, and so forth that use animals and are filmed in North America are required to give the AHA full access to their sets (*Humane Hollywood* 2018c). However, films that are not part of the SAG are under no obligation to follow the AHA's guidelines if they do not wish to (*Humane Hollywood* 2018c). If a non-SAG film chooses not to follow the AHA's guidelines, all this means is that they will not be eligible for any of the AHA's disclaimers.

independent group with no conflict of interest (*American Humane* 2019f). They currently monitor around 70% of professional American film sets, which is around 2000 productions annually (*American Humane* 2019f). However, in 2013, *The Hollywood Reporter* released a detailed exposé that questioned the AHA's practices and ethics, concluding that they are "inadequate" (Baum 2013a).[17]

The AHA is notable for their "No animals were harmed…" slogan, which was first used in 1972 on *The Doberman Gang* (*American Humane* 2019d). Since then, it has become a reassuring disclaimer for film audiences worldwide (*Humane Hollywood* 2018e). As this book has demonstrated elsewhere, the use of animals is much more socially-acceptable when it is hidden, attenuated, or romanticized. This can be achieved through reassuring labels, such as "free range" or "no animals were harmed". However, the AHA's seal of approval has evidently been allotted to films that have entailed potentially harmful incidents involving animals, such as *A Dog's Purpose*.[18] This is because a film can still receive the disclaimer even if an animal was harmed or killed as long as the film was following the AHA's guidelines when the incident occurred. For example, *Life of Pi* (2012) was awarded the "No animals were harmed" disclaimer, even though there was strong evidence to suggest that a tiger nearly drowned during filming (Child 2013; Baum 2013b). Only films rated as "Outstanding" are permitted to use the full "No animals were harmed…" disclaimer.[19] However, since 99.98% of AHA-monitored films achieve the "outstanding" rating, many have questioned just how strict the AHA

---

[17] This detailed *exposé* interviewed six AHA staff members and reviewed a large amount of internal AHA documents, such as logs, e-mails, and meeting minutes. The article claimed that the AHA "distorts its film ratings, downplays or fails to publicly acknowledge harmful incidents and sometimes does not seriously pursue investigations" (Baum 2013a).

[18] Since *A Dog's Purpose* was a SAG production, the use of animals on-set had been monitored by the AHA throughout filming (*BBC News* 2017). However, the AHA's independent investigation of the leaked video, which was swiftly completed in just over two weeks, concluded that the footage was "misleading" and "manipulated" (*American Humane* 2019e). Furthermore, the AHA's official statement did not condemn the actions of those involved in the incident, but instead questioned the "motives and ethics" of whomever leaked the footage. The AHA concluded their investigation by stating that: "No animals were harmed in the making of this film" (*American Humane* 2019e).

[19] There are currently six different grades given by the AHA: 1. Monitored: Outstanding, 2. Monitored: Acceptable, 3. Monitored: Special Circumstances, 4. Monitored: Unacceptable, 5. Not Monitored: Production Compliant, and 6. Not Monitored (*Humane Hollywood* 2018c).

are when assigning these grades (*PR Newswire* 2013). The AHA is allowed to view scripts before filming, and the AHA's set monitors can show up on-set at any time during the filming of any scene involving animals (Baum 2013a). Whether or not a film can receive the AHA's disclaimer is decided once a production is finished. Once the final edit of a film is complete, it is viewed by the AHA to ensure that the scenes involving animals were the same ones that the AHA's set monitor viewed (*Humane Hollywood* 2018b). However, this means that the AHA only judges the welfare of animals physically on-set (*American Humane* 2019f). They do not assess the welfare of any animals in training, transit, or holding, which is, as Part 1 demonstrated, where animals are more likely to experience mistreatment or neglect. The AHA even admits that some of their "outstanding" or "acceptable" films may have entailed animal deaths, but they insist that in these cases the animal's death was off-set and/or not the fault of the production company or the AHA (Baum 2013a). Thus, the AHA essentially masks problems that follow from using animals for performance rather than tackling the core issues with using animals as performers. Since 1997, the AHA's set monitors have been licensed law enforcement officers within the state of California. This means that they can write citations and even make arrests. Nevertheless, the AHA is yet to use either of these legal powers, even though they are estimated to have monitored over 35,000 films in this time (Baum 2013a).

There are over 500 points made in the AHA's 131-page guideline book. For example: on-set sedation is banned, except in veterinary emergencies (*American Humane* 2019c). The introduction of the guidebook claims that:

> At its most fundamental level, American Humane Association's role is to prevent legally defined cruelty to animal actors. In reality, the industry today is primarily composed of ***caring and responsible*** individuals. (*American Humane* 2019c) [emphasis added]

This statement seems somewhat naïve given that there were many instances of intentional harm towards animals before the AHA began monitoring film sets. Moreover, it seems to imply support for, and thus bias towards, the industry that the AHA claims to be impartial towards.

The AHA's claims of impartiality are further questionable when considered alongside their response to incidents involving animal harm. To illustrate, after the controversy surrounding *A Dog's Purpose*, the AHA did not condemn the actions of those who allegedly forced Hercules underwater. Instead, they criticized the person(s) who released the footage (*American Humane* 2019e). This suggests, along with the AHA's guidebook introduction, that the AHA is not entirely impartial.

Disney has a strong working relationship with the AHA that began in the 1940s and continues to the present day (*The Official Disney Fan Club* 2018). To illustrate, in 1955, the AHA awarded Walt with a plaque to celebrate his "humane ideals". The plaque is displayed at the main *Disneyland* theme park (Strodder 2015: 21). The AHA has proudly monitored hundreds of live-action Disney films and television shows, even in countries where the AHA has no jurisdiction. For example, the AHA monitored *102 Dalmatians* (2000), which was filmed in London (Frammalino and Bates 2001). Given that the AHA has a strong reputation for good animal welfare, Disney's association with them suggests that Disney is keen to associate their films with the good treatment of animal actors. Similarly, in 2008, WDAS released Bolt, a film centred around the ethics of using live animals in the film industry.

Bolt is a CGI-animated WDAS film about the ethics of using animals, particularly dogs, as actors in the film industry. Bolt, the film's protagonist, is a canine actor that "stars" in a live-action television show. However, he does not understand the difference between his reality and his role in the television show. He believes that he has the life, relationships, and super-powers of the superhero dog character that he portrays. At the beginning of the film, Bolt is chosen as a puppy from an animal shelter by Penny (his human co-star). Soon after, they are seen starring in a television show (also named *Bolt*) together. However, at the end of each day of filming, Bolt stays on-set in a trailer, whereas (unbeknownst to him) Penny and the other animal actors go home to their real lives.

Throughout the film it is clear that both Bolt and Penny want to live together off-set; however, they are prohibited from doing so by the television producers and Penny's agent. This is because the producers place much importance on Bolt's belief that the television show is real. This decision is portrayed as being harmful towards both Bolt and Penny.

Early in the film, Penny asks her mother and agent (Roland) if she can take Bolt home:

Penny: So I can bring Bolt home?
Roland: As your friend I say, "Yes, absolutely," but as your agent, I have to remind you this is Bolt's world. He has to stay right here. Okay, let's go.
Penny: But he never gets to be a real dog, and it would only be for the weekend…

Bolt and Penny's forced separation is at the forefront of this film; it is presented as the worst harm that Bolt routinely experiences as an animal actor. Moreover, Bolt appears to be the only actor this harm applies to. The television show Bolt stars in also features two cats, both of which leave the set each night. These two cats enjoy verbally taunting Bolt about his beliefs that the show is real. Thus, the cats do know that the show is not real, which Bolt does not. When compared to some of the ways that animal actors have been treated by the film industry, such as the treatment of horses during the filming of *Jesse James* (1939), the treatment of animal actors in *Bolt* does not seem particularly harmful. Bolt is never physically mistreated or badly neglected by the film industry. It is more that as an animal actor his life is severely restricted in a way that he is unable to fully-understand. He lives in a trailer on-set and is apparently only allowed to leave when filming scenes. However, it is notable that he is lives in a clean, spacious, nicely-decorated trailer, not a cage. Thus, even though *Bolt* acknowledges that the freedom of animal performers is restricted, Bolt is still presented as living comfortably. This is in stark contrast to how animal actors have been treated by the film industry in reality. Therefore, WDAS is again only exploring instances of mild animal harm that are easily-resolved. This was also highlighted in the previous chapter with regards to pet-ownership in *Lady and the Tramp*.

The film ends with Bolt and Penny getting what they wished for throughout the film; in the film's final scene, Bolt is seen living comfortably in Penny's home after they both retire from the entertainment industry. However, it should be added that Bolt's happy ending (retiring from entertainment and living with his human co-star) is not unrealistic. Research has found that many domesticated animal actors do live in permanent homes off-set, rather than shelters and the like (Wills 2012). For example, the "dire wolves" in *Game of Thrones* (2011–2019) were portrayed by Northern-Inuit dogs that lived with the show's actors off-set when not working (Vonledebur 2013). The AHA has even noted and praised films in which this has happened, such as *Pirates of the Caribbean: The Curse of the Black Pearl* (2003) (*Humane Hollywood* 2018f). Thus, WDAS is depicting an issue that rarely affects dog actors. As evidenced in Part I, wild animals usually end up in zoos and shelters once they retire from performance. This is perhaps why WDAS chose to make *Bolt* about a domesticated animal performer rather than a wild one.[20] If WDAS had centred *Bolt* around a wild animal actor, it would have been unrealistic to have given them an ending in which they either lived with a human off-set or were allowed back into their natural environment. Therefore, the ending of *Bolt* is only believable with domestic animals. As highlighted in Part III, Disney's recent re-make of *Dumbo* (2019) did feature such an ending; however, this was apparently only after campaigns from animal welfare organizations. If there had been no campaigns for this romantic ending, perhaps it would never have materialized. As highlighted in Part I, the lives animal performers have after entertainment is one of the main problems with using animals for this purpose. In both versions of *Dumbo* (1941) (2019), plus *Bolt* (2008), this is not portrayed as a problem; in every one of these narratives, the animal protagonist gets the life they desire. Yet in reality, this ending can only realistically happen to domestic animals.

As well as minimizing the harms animal actors can experience in the film industry, *Bolt* romanticizes some aspects of the film industry. For example, it is Bolt (the dog), not Penny (the human), who is the star of the television show. To illustrate, the promotional material for the television show (depicted within the narrative) focusses upon Bolt rather than Penny. On Bolt's journey back to Hollywood, he is recognised by other animals, which greatly aids him. For example, Bolt becomes friends with Rhino the hamster after Rhino recognises Bolt. This friendship helps Bolt find his way back to Hollywood. Thus, *Bolt* seems to acknowledge the value that animal performers can bring to television shows and films. However, it suggests that the animals themselves can benefit significantly from this fame, even though this is unlikely to be the case in reality.

[20] *Bolt* is not based upon any external texts; it was devised by WDAS (IMDB 2017).

Bolt does imply that film sets can be dangerous locations, but only accidentally. The introduction of the film features Bolt and Penny filming a "chase scene", which includes many risky stunts. For example, Bolt is required to run swiftly between moving traffic as he is stalked by masked humans on motorbike. These scenes are filmed without danger. However, the film ends with a near-fatal fire (caused accidentally by props) that almost kills Penny. It is in this scene that Bolt demonstrates his undying loyalty to Penny by heroically saving her from the fire. Bolt is initially outdoors during the fire, and thus safe, but he runs inside to save Penny. Yet because it is an *accidental* fire that almost kills Penny and Bolt, the film industry is somewhat blameless here. Moreover, it is a human (Penny) that is severely injured in the fire, not an animal. In reality, the dangers that animal performers face are usually part of filmmaking/shows and thus purposeful, not accidental. This was true of the harms faced by animals in both *Jesse James* and *A Dog's Purpose*, for example. Thus, like *Dumbo* and *Bongo*, *Bolt* is both a romantic, simplified, portrayal of the entertainment industry. It acknowledges that film sets can be harmful towards animals, but only minimally or accidentally. Film sets are not depicted as locations in which animals experience purposeful or malicious harms, even though this has sometimes been the case in reality.

At the end of *Bolt*, both Bolt and Penny are replaced in their television show by new human and dog actors. Thus, the fictional television show in *Bolt* continues to be in production and continues to use animals. The dog that replaces Bolt does not speak, nor is it given an individual name. Thus, it is less-anthropomorphised and individualized than Bolt is. This instinctively makes the welfare of this nameless dog less-concerning to audiences. Additionally, the villainous cat actors that torment Bolt early in the film presumably also keep their role in the show. As the previous chapter demonstrated, villainous animals are often punished for their anti-social behaviour, which may be why the fate of these cat actors is not returned to. Thus, even though the film criticizes the use of animal actors, the film ends with animal actors continuing to be used in the film industry without criticism. Thus, the message of *Bolt* seems to be that only individualized, named, anthropomorphised, pro-social, animals should not have to perform, if this is their choice. Additionally, in *Bolt*, animal actors (including Bolt for the most part) are happy and willing to perform. Bolt's unhappiness is not because he is an actor; he is unhappy because he is abruptly separated from Penny (which happens outside of filming). Thus, as with *Dumbo*, animals are portrayed as wanting, and even happy, to perform for humans.

To summarize, the six problems with making animals perform (as highlighted in Part I) are not meaningfully considered in *Bolt*. Firstly, Bolt is depicted as wanting to perform; at no point is he depicted as being trained to perform in harsh conditions. Secondly, Bolt's performance is based around his natural abilities as a dog (such as running fast); he is not performing human-like behaviours or made to dress in human clothing. Thirdly, Bolt's living conditions are adequate; he lives in a roomy trailer and appears to be well cared for. It is only his loneliness that is an issue for him, which is fully-resolved at the end of the film. Fourthly, once Bolt retires from the film industry, he is allowed to live permanently with his human co-star. Thus, he does not end up living in a shelter or similar. Fifthly, Bolt poses no danger to humans; in fact, he wishes to protect them rather than harm them. Sixthly, Bolt is respected by many of the humans involved in film-making. For example, by not allowing Bolt to be fully-aware on the reality of his life, the producers seem to acknowledge that Bolt is sentient and can think for himself. Thus, he is not metaphorically objectified, which many animal actors are in reality. In summary, the six main issues with using animals for performance are not depicted in *Bolt*. They are replaced by much-simpler issues, all of which are harmoniously resolved by the end of the film. Moreover, the main issue Bolt experiences (living on-set) is not usually an issue for Bolt's species. Additionally, the film does not depict Bolt being removed from his mother, living most of his life caged, being mutilated, or being trained with violence. Yet these harms are commonly experienced by animals in the entertainment industry. Thus, the film ignores the true problems animal performers experience and instead depicts highly-unlikely scenarios, such as Bolt being accidently shipped across North America.

One of the most unrealistic aspects of *Bolt* is perhaps that the AHA is not depicted or even mentioned. This is unusual given that they are such a significant part of the professional American film industry, which the narrative is set in. However, since *Bolt* expresses sympathy towards animal actors, if it had included the AHA, it would have been challenging to have depicted them favourably. There is little in *Bolt* that the AHA would take exception to. As a result, if the events if *Bolt* were to happen on the set of a real television show, that show would still be awarded the AHA's "No animals were harmed…" disclaimer. Such a depiction, whilst realistic, would surely be classed as a negative portrayal of the AHA. As highlighted earlier, the AHA is only concerned with legal, on-set, animal harm. Thus, there is nothing within *Bolt* that the AHA would object to. As evidenced earlier, Disney has had a strong working relationship with the AHA for many years. Thus, the AHA's existence was likely entirely removed to avoid any portrayals that could have jeopardized this relationship. Yet, as highlighted in Chap. 2, *Brother Bear* (a film set long before the film industry existed) gently mocks the AHA's "no animals were harmed" slogan at the end of the film. Thus, WDAS has referenced, and joked about, the AHA previously; however, it was in a film far removed from the AHA's normal context, and thus far from potential scrutiny.

Conclusion

Bolt and *Dumbo* (1941) are both animated films. In fact, the majority of Disney films that oppose using or harming animals are animated. For example, *Bambi* and *The Fox and The Hound* are both films that oppose harming animals, and they are both animations. This suggests that while Disney is keen to release films that condemn harming animals, they are much more likely to do it in animated form. Additionally, Disney's recent live-action films, such as *The Jungle Book* (2016) and *The Lion King* (2019), have been produced with CGI animals; thus, no "animal actors" were used at all. The evidence presented in this chapter suggests that the use of animals for entertainment is becoming socially-unacceptable. This is because animal performers are usually higher-order individualized animals that are visible. As a result, there are significant changes occurring for the benefit of animal performers. However, these changes are not originating from the AHA or any legal system, they are mostly arising from campaigns and shifts in public perceptions. For example, Disney no longer uses ape actors; this is likely because of the increasing public backlash towards this practice. It would be perfectly legal for Disney to continue using apes, yet to do so in the face of negative public perceptions of this practice would surely damage the company's animal-friendly reputation. Further to this, the message of several recent Disney films has further suggested that Disney is objecting to the use of animals in entertainment and captivity. For example, *Dumbo* (2019) ends with the captive animals being freed, and the circus that held them vowing never to use animals for entertainment again. These points suggest that Disney is taking the stance that using live animals for performance is unacceptable.

6

Conclusion

Walt was somewhat bemused by the intense academic analysis his work received. For example, he famously stated that: "We make the pictures and then let the professors tell us what they mean" (in: Fleming 2016: 195). Thus, it is unlikely that he would have thought highly of this book or its conclusions. However, this text has not been about Walt, nor is it only about WDAS films or even Disney. This book has been principally concerned with how animal harm and objectification have been depicted in cultural representations, and WDAS films have been used to exemplify that case. Ultimately, this book has demonstrated that whether or not animal harm is depicted as socially-acceptable in mainstream cultural representations depends upon four factors: the species affected, the number of animals involved, the social-acceptance of the harm, and the visibility of that harm.

Depictions of animals, and the products created from their bodies, are widespread within cultural representations, such as WDAS films. However, very few texts have questioned how WDAS has depicted the harms that many animals experience even though those harms are frequently implicated in WDAS's films. For example, WDAS films often depict meat and farm animals, yet they have never depicted a slaughterhouse (the process by which farm animals unwillingly "become" meat). Thus, previous scholars have questioned what is included in WDAS's

R. R. Stanton, *The Disneyfication of Animals*, The Palgrave Macmillan Animal Ethics Series, https://doi.org/10.1007/978-3-030-49316-5_6

depictions, but very few have questioned what WDAS has *excluded*. This omission is important because three billion animals are legally killed every day, yet these animals—their lives, deaths, and the harms entailed by mankind's use of animals—are seldom depicted in mainstream cultural representations (of which WDAS films are a key example). Thus, it is clear that this text has a significant place within both Disney and animal studies.

Humans are one of 8.7 million animal species on Earth, yet humans routinely treat other animals in ways that entail causing harm and death on massive scales (Black 2011). Simultaneously, cultural representations, such as WDAS films, routinely minimise those harms or romanticize human-animal relationships. Culturally, the scale of harms done to animals remains invisible, and that helps to normalize the status quo wherein animals are harmed. As a major media conglomerate that routinely depicts human-animal interactions in films that are seen by millions, if not billions, of viewers, WDAS has a significant global influence. WDAS films imply that some species, such as dogs, should be treated with respect and never harmed. However, they also perpetuate the idea that other species, such as fish, are not worthy of respect. Cumulatively, WDAS has helped to sustain a cultural imbalance that normalizes speciesist attitudes and negates the real harms that characterize human-animal relationships in the real world. For many people, cultural representations provide the only experience they have with many species of animals, particularly wild or exotic animals. Therefore, if these representations are false or misleading, it may affect how millions of people view that species in reality. As this book has shown, this point is demonstrated by the "Disney effect" and "*Jaws* effect", for example. Additionally, while people are unaware or mis-educated about the realities of using animals, the situation is unlikely to improve for the animals involved. As highlighted in Chaps. 1 and 5, practical changes in animal welfare are caused by exposing the reality of how animals are treated by the industries that use them. Thus, if cultural representations attenuate the harms animals experience, these issues are unlikely to be resolved.

Animal harm and objectification are more widespread than they have been at any previous juncture in history. The negative effects of this situation are not limited to animals; they also impact upon humans and the environment. However, that situation in itself does not explain why Disney specifically should care about their depictions of animals and the harms that animals face. Speciesist attitudes are not exclusively perpetuated via WDAS films; such attitudes are commonly iterated in mainstream Anglo-American cultural representations, including WDAS's filmic rivals. As the chapters of this book have demonstrated, the public are rarely encouraged to reflect upon speciesism, and speciesist attitudes are rarely challenged in mainstream culture. However, as producers of cultural representations, WDAS has the unique potential to shape the discourses surrounding perceptions of animals and animal welfare. It has been proposed that Disney can influence behavioural changes that impact on animal welfare. For example, sales of fur hats massively increased during the Davy Crockett era, and hunting as an activity declined after *Bambi*. Furthermore, the "Disney effect" demonstrates the direct power companies like Disney have over which species and breeds of animals are chosen as pets, and even how they are treated. Very few other organizations have this powerful global impact. Thus, Disney *should* consider how they depict animals, and the harms animals experience, because there is much research to suggest that their portrayals of animals and animal harm can affect animals in reality, which is not true of most other companies.

The fact that all WDAS films are suitable for children further emphasizes why WDAS's depictions of animals warrant study. Disney has a fundamental role in modern American culture that involves them being trusted to teach children moral codes about what is pro-social and anti-social (Wills 2017: 106). Children often experience animals through cultural representations, yet they are rarely taught or informed about the harsh realities of how animals are treated. Children are mostly presented with misleading romantic images that fail to depict the harms inflicted upon animals or the massive scale of those harms. Because of this, children (in the Anglo-American context) are unaware that their lifestyles are indirectly supporting industries that harm, objectify, and, in many cases kill, animals. The partial picture children receive about animal welfare—which almost entirely negates the routine harms done to animals—is likely to skew how children think about these issues.

In animation (and cel animation in particular), every scene, character, and detail is painstakingly crafted. Thus, every animal in every WDAS film was designed with purpose, and thus every instance of objectification or speciesism was intentional (strictly speaking).[1] There is strong evidence that WDAS's outputs are shaped by broader shifts in socially-normative attitudes. Some of WDAS's early films contain representations that are no longer socially-acceptable. In some cases, WDAS has even attempted to retrospectively "correct" past depictions that are no longer considered socially-acceptable. For example, "Sunflower", the human-donkey hybrid in 1941's *Fantasia*, has been completely removed from modern edits of *Fantasia* as she represents a derogatory racist stereotype that is now unacceptable.[2] Furthermore, Disney does not appear to even reference Sunflower's existence even though Disney still promotes *Fantasia*. Thus, it is clear that WDAS has consciously attempted to alter their depictions of race, gender, religion, and so forth to align with prevailing contemporaneous social attitudes. Yet, even though WDAS has consciously attempted to stop portraying humans in discriminatory ways, they continue to portray animals in discriminatory ways. This book has repeatedly demonstrated that WDAS films imply that higher-order species, particularly those that are neotenous, named, individualized, anthropomorphised, or pro-social should be treated better than non-anthropomorphised, nameless, lower-order species. Thus, WDAS films have repeatedly reflected socially-acceptable speciesist attitudes from 1937 until 2016. This is a problem because speciesism is just as problematic and harmful as sexism, racism, and other forms of discrimination because it is responsible for billions of deaths every day.

Despite the severity of speciesism, there are few signs that WDAS is attempting to seriously challenge their speciesist attitudes. One of WDAS's most recent films, *Zootopia* (2016), indicates that speciesist attitudes are morally wrong. *Zootopia* is set in a world populated by anthropomorphised mammals. These animals live and work alongside each

[1] It is unclear to what extent the animators are unconsciously replicating social norms, or to what extent those representations are designed to appeal to the broadest possible demographic by reflecting normative ideas about animals.

[2] Further information on Sunflower, and her removal from modern releases of *Fantasia* (1940), can be found in: Murguía 2018: 180–182.

other in the city of Zootopia. However, some species exhibit speciesist attitudes towards other species. For example, many of the characters hold the opinion that foxes are trouble-makers and sheep are gentle. As the film progresses, it becomes clear that these attitudes are problematic because every animal in the city of Zootopia has an individual personality. Thus, the message of the film is that speciesism is logically and morally wrong. However, there is not one bird or fish species in *Zootopia*'s all-animal cast. Therefore, birds and fish are excluded from the film's apparent anti-speciesist message. Given that fish and birds are the most-common victims of speciesism in reality, and that those harms are underpinned by speciesist attitudes, their exclusion from *Zootopia* is problematic.[3] If this film sought to proffer an anti-speciesist message, a more inclusive approach to its depictions of different species would have solidified that message. As a result, *Zootopia*, a film about the ethical objections to speciesism, inadvertently reinforces speciesist attitudes. Thus, even WDAS's criticism of speciesism is speciesist.

Throughout this book, there have been several points made in relation to animal studies and Disney studies. Those points will now be summarized in conclusion of this text.

How Are Animal Harm and Objectification Depicted in WDAS Films (1937–2016)?

WDAS repeatedly romanticizes, humourizes, and minimizes the routine harm and objectification commonly experienced by animals in reality. To illustrate, WDAS's vision of farming is limited to small, independent, free-range farms. The norms of industrialised factory farming (the second most-common killer of animals globally) are absent from WDAS's body of films. WDAS's romanticization and minimization of animal harm is further illustrated by the optimism and hope evident in situations of animal harm. The number of animals that escape the routine harm and

[3] As demonstrated in Chap. 2, fish are the most-common victims of routine animal harm in terms of numbers. Similarly, as demonstrated in Chap. 1, chickens are the most common victims of factory farming (which is the second most-common killer of animals globally). Thus, fish and birds are the most common victims of speciesism in terms of numbers.

objectification assigned to their species in reality is so low that it is almost-always newsworthy when it does happen. This was evidenced by the emotive reaction to Phoenix, the calf who survived death twice during the UK's foot-and-mouth outbreak (Browne 2001). [4] However, the number of animals slaughtered in reality is so high that it could never be accurately known and has to be roughly estimated to the nearest billion. Yet in WDAS films, the opposite logic is true. The number of times animals die or face serious harm in WDAS films is minimal, yet it is commonplace for higher-order, anthropomorphised, species to escape from harmful situations in WDAS films. Thus, WDAS is depicting the hopeful, romantic opposite of animal harm. In short, WDAS films that feature animal harm usually have optimism and luck, but reality does not. However, this point is only true of animals that are anthropomorphised, neotenous, pro-social, higher-order, and/or individualized.

Further to this, WDAS mostly challenges animal welfare issues that are easily resolved. To illustrate, *Lady and the Tramp* focusses upon simple issues commonly experienced by pets, such as a lack of dog license. The more serious issues pets routinely experience are either minimized or ignored by the narrative. Additionally, WDAS has only challenged animal welfare issues that are already socially-unacceptable or becoming socially-unacceptable. For example, although WDAS questioned the ethics of killing puppies to create fur clothing in *Dalmatians*, they have never addressed the ethics of killing cows to produce leather, which is a much more socially-acceptable and common practice. Thus, WDAS is selective with the animal welfare issues that they will question. As highlighted in Chap. 5, the use of animals in entertainment has become socially-unacceptable. This is perhaps why this industry has rarely been depicted by WDAS. On the few occasions when animal performers have been portrayed, a small amount of the harms they can experience have been

[4] During the UK's outbreak of foot-and-mouth disease in 2001, a single calf (Phoenix) became famous after surviving death twice. Phoenix had been given the lethal injection, along with 70 other cattle and 47 sheep. However, she was found alive, buried under the other animal carcasses, six days later. Despite the severity of the foot-and-mouth crisis, it was decided that Phoenix would not be killed again (Browne 2001). This was likely because of the high-profile campaigns, such as the one by *The Mirror* newspaper, that pleaded for her to be saved from death (Browne 2001). This high-profile instance involving a singular, named, farm animal demonstrates how rare it is that a farm animal escapes the routine harm assigned to their species.

highlighted. However, the harms that the animals in these films experience are always happily resolved by the end of the film. Thus, the worst harms that the animals used by these industries experience are ignored by WDAS even though the industries themselves are challenged. Additionally, when attitudes towards industries that use animals change, Disney changes their stance. To illustrate, Disney's recent re-make of *Dumbo* changed the 1941 ending to one more in line with contemporary attitudes towards captive animals. In these ways, WDAS and Disney films reflect how socially-acceptable contemporaneous forms of animal harm and objectification are at any moment in Anglo-American culture.

This text has looked specifically at the harms animals experience from humans, or as a result of humans. It has been clear that WDAS's human characters who harm pro-social animals are usually portrayed villainously. Specifically, there are two types of villain: the intriguing and the repellent (Forbes 2011: 13–27). The intriguing villain is a character such as Cruella (*Dalmatians*) or Alameda Slim (*Home on the Range*). These intriguing villains often plan to harm animals, yet they usually fail in comical circumstances. To illustrate, Cruella is comically outwitted by the many Dalmatian puppies she wishes to make a fur coat from. It is vital that the aims of the intriguing villains are unsuccessful for their character to remain engaging and thus memorable. Despite being villainous and trying to repeatedly harm animals, such characters are often remembered fondly. For example, Cruella De Vil, is undoubtedly one of WDAS's most revered characters, villainous or otherwise, despite her murderous intentions. In contrast to the intriguing villain, WDAS's repellent villains are notorious for their lack of remorse. Such characters, such as the faceless hunters in *Bambi*, are rarer. Moreover, they are not remembered fondly. To illustrate, the repellent hunters in *Bambi* feature in no known Disney merchandise. These repellent villains are rarer because there are limits to WDAS's depictions of animal harm. Despite the prevalence of animals in WDAS films, animals rarely die or are seriously harmed in WDAS films. When humans attempt to harm animals, the animals almost-always escape. This is again because WDAS is hopeful towards situations of animal harm. Most of the humans that attempt to directly harm higher-order, neotenous, anthropomorphised animals in WDAS films are unsuccessful. Moreover, they are usually villainous characters, which means that harming, or attempting to harm, certain types of animals is depicted as an anti-social behaviour in WDAS films.

Additionally, in many cases the harms animals experience are caused by other animals. For example, in *Cinderella*, it is Lucifer the cat who tries to harm the mice. The mice are actually protected and saved from harm by Cinderella (who is human). In other instances, animals face harm as a result of their own actions and decisions. For example, in *Home on the Range*, the dairy cows face no harm on their beloved dairy farm, but much harm after they decide to leave it at their own free will. Therefore, in contrast to reality, humans are often not to blame for animal harm in WDAS films. In fact, humans that help animals are usually pro-social characters. Thus, WDAS presents animal harm as anti-social and kindness towards animals as pro-social. Therefore, direct animal harm is depicted as a socially-unacceptable behaviour in WDAS films.

How Have Different Animal Species Been Depicted in WDAS Films?

This text has demonstrated that WDAS films reflect how commonplace speciesist attitudes are. WDAS films consistently suggest that higher-order, individualized, neotenous, heavily-anthropomorphised, pro-social mammals do not deserve to experience routine harm or discrimination. In fact, higher-order species are treated more favourably than some demographics of humans. For example, elderly women and Native Americans are just two of the many demographics that have often been depicted in a derogatory manner in WDAS films.[5] In regards to animals, pet dogs are almost-always depicted favourably. However, lower-order species, such as birds, fish, and working animals are usually objectified (either metaphorically or literally). As characters, they are mostly non-anthropomorphised, genderless, nameless, and so forth. WDAS uses these animals to add realism, context, or decoration. This bias implies

---

[5] For further information on how Disney has repeatedly depicted certain demographics of humans in derogatory ways, see *Diversity in Disney Films: Critical Essays on Race, Ethnicity, Gender, Sexuality and Disability* edited by Johnson Cheu (2013).

that WDAS does not consider these species to be as worthy of attention as their higher-order, mostly mammalian, counterparts.

Additionally, lower-order species, such as fish and insects, experience normalized harm and objectification, which WDAS's narratives encourage little sympathy for. There is no solemn music or pained reaction from the other characters when a non-anthropomorphised, lower-order, species is harmed or even killed. For example, in *Fantasia 2000*, hundreds of fish are pulled from the sea by a net. They are then boxed-up and sold on land. Thus, they certainly die. However, the narrative only encourages sympathy for an anthropomorphised toy soldier that has accidently got lost between these fish, rather than the fish themselves.

There are two common exceptions to this point. First, villainous higher-order animals, such as Lucifer the cat (*Cinderella*) or Iago the parrot (*Aladdin*), usually face harm or death for which their narrative offers no sympathy. However, such incidents occur at the end of their narrative, after they have established themselves as antagonistic by trying to harm (or even kill) pro-social characters. Therefore, the subsequent harm or misfortune that they experience is depicted as deserved rather than cruel. The second exception is that lower-order species that are heavily-anthropomorphised are usually spared harm. For example, in *Brother Bear*, the only salmon that is not harmed is the anthropomorphised, individualized one that appears at the end of the film in a joke about the AHA. Therefore, anthropomorphism and behaviour, as well as species, dictates whether or not an animal character will experience socially-acceptable harm.

Why Have Different Forms of Animal Harm or Objectification Been Depicted with Differing Levels of Sympathy?

This question is partly answered by the previous point; higher-order, neotenized, anthropomorphised species are offered more sympathy than lower-order species when they experience harm. This is also true of reality. For instance, as Chap. 5 evidenced, there have been many campaigns to improve the welfare of individual, higher-order, animals in captivity (for example: *PETA* 2019b, d, o). However, there is another key reason why different forms of harm and objectification are depicted in different ways: the number of animals involved. Every chapter of this book has demonstrated that the "collapse of compassion" effect significantly affects people's reactions towards animal harm. People almost-always express more concern for issues that affect individual or small numbers of animals. Furthermore, WDAS only challenges issues that affect a small number of animals, such as the entertainment industry. The industries that kill the most animals (fish farming and factory farming) have never been depicted, or even referenced, by WDAS. Moreover, these issues are often ignored by animal rights' campaigners, as Chap. 2 evidenced with fishing. Further to this, WDAS films individualize the animal characters that they want the audience to develop sympathy towards, such as pet mammals. For example, before Lady the dog (*Lady and the Tramp*) experiences harm, the narrative establishes her as an individual, pro-social, character that deserves respect. Therefore, her mistreatment and misfortune seems more tragic as a result. In contrast, WDAS's birds, fish, and working animals are typically presented in large homogenous, non-anthropomorphised, groups. When such groups are harmed en-masse, the "collapse of compassion" response is elicited, and empathy for the individuals comprising the group is inhibited. For example, in *Mulan* (1998), an avalanche kills many warriors on horseback, yet the narrative encourages no sympathy for the many warriors or their horses. In contrast, the death of a singular deer (in *Bambi*) is one of WDAS's most famously emotive moments. Thus, the welfare of large groups of characters is less-concerning to audiences in such scenarios, even though a far greater number of animals are harmed. In summary, WDAS depicts the harm experienced by higher-order, neotenous, anthropomorphised, *individualized* animals as being more concerning than harms that affect lower-order, non-anthropomorphised, *grouped* animals. Therefore, the "collapse of compassion" effect is not exclusive to humans or to reality; it also applies to animated fictional animals. Moreover, Disney is using this reaction to their advantage.

Can Depictions of Animals and Animal Harm/ Objectification Affect Species in Reality?

The technological developments since 1937 (the release of *Snow White*) have had both positive and negative effects on the treatment of animals worldwide. For example, as Chap. 1 demonstrated, the technological advancements in farm machinery have made life much worse for many species of farm animals. In contrast, technological advancements in the film industry have changed animal performance for the better by enabling film companies to use CGI rather than animal performers. This means that the film industry is no longer using as many animals as they would have previously; thus, less animal performers are experiencing the harms associated with the film industry. However, film technology is not the only way that film is improving the treatment of animals. This book has demonstrated that the message of films can encourage practical changes towards animals in reality. WDAS's animal-centred films, such as *Dumbo*, *Bambi*, *Dalmatians*, and others, have evidently improved animal welfare through their message. This can also be seen with non-WDAS, animal-centred, films, such as *Babe* (1995). However, in most cases, this was not the primary purpose of those films. In contrast to this, several films produced with the sole purpose of improving animal welfare, such as *Earthlings* (2005), *Dominion* (2018), and the many PETA exposés, have had far fewer viewings than most WDAS films. To illustrate, Box Office Mojo, a website that documents how much revenue a film takes, does not even list *Earthlings* or *Dominion* in their database. This suggests that both films had low-revenue and thus few viewings. In comparison, WDAS films are known for being hugely-profitable and watched by millions of viewers (Wasko 2001: 252). Thus, people are more likely to develop their opinions of animals and animal harm from WDAS films. Documentaries such as *Earthlings* are notoriously difficult to engage with because of their violent imagery and tone of despair (for example, see: Sullivan 2017). In contrast, the WDAS films that encouraged a change in attitude towards animals have been romantic, optimistic, and comedic rather than violent and hopeless. For example, *Dalmatians*, a film about the ethics of producing fur clothing, features very little violence towards animals and no animal deaths at all. In fact, most of the violence in *Dalmatians* is directed towards humans. Additionally, every would-be victim of the fur industry avoids their fate in *Dalmatians*. Thus, the film offers a very romantic and optimistic portrayal of the notoriously cruel and violent fur industry. Despite this lack of realism, its message worked. After the release of *Dalmatians*, sales of fur products significantly declined. Similarly, as highlighted in Chap. 3, PETA's most influential campaigns have been those that avoided violent or bloody imagery, such as their "We'd rather go naked than wear fur" campaign. This demonstrates that non-violent campaigns and films appear to be more engaging and successful than confrontational (albethey realistic) ones. Thus, since they are characteristically romantic, comedic, and optimistic texts, WDAS films have the potential to challenge assumptions about animal welfare issues while still engaging with viewers and being financially and critically successful. WDAS films are aimed towards broad family demographics, and realistic depictions of animal harm, such as those that occur in industrialised farming, have the potential to be upsetting. However, WDAS has managed to balance these issues on occasion. For example, the terrifying hunting in *Bambi* was a small part of a much larger text that also contained humour, romance, and other palatable elements, making it still an enjoyable and entertaining film despite its darker tones. Even today, more than seventy years after it was first released, *Bambi* is still cited as a film that passionately demonstrates why hunting is immoral. Moreover, merchandise from this film is still widely produced and sold today. This suggests that the anti-hunting message of *Bambi* was successful, but so too were the romantic elements.

WDAS produces animated features, and their main aims as a company are to entertain and to generate profit. As such, WDAS does not have a direct responsibility towards animals in the same way that PETA (whose mandate is to help animals) does. This book has been fairly critical of WDAS's romanticism and lack of realism. However, despite the flaws in WDAS's romanticism, WDAS's approach to story-telling might be a useful way to engage audiences to reflect upon animal welfare issues. Therefore, WDAS's romantic approach offers animal welfare organizations an effective way into successfully opposing animal harm and objectification. Thus, organizations such as PETA should adopt the approach that has evidently been so effective for WDAS; they should challenge animal welfare issues with romance, humour, and optimism, rather than violent imagery. However, given that Disney's influence has not always benefitted animals, caution is needed here. To illustrate, it is claimed that the "Disney effect" has negatively affected many breeds of dogs. Thus, it would be beneficial for organizations such as PETA to work closely with companies, such as WDAS, to have positive impacts on animal welfare and to avoid potential negative impacts. In summary, WDAS's approach to challenging animal harm and objectification could be beneficial to animal welfare campaigners, but that approach must be practiced cautiously.

What Does WDAS's Depiction of Harm Towards Animals Reveal About Violence in WDAS Films Generally?

It has often been argued that there is too much violence in the media, and in WDAS films specifically (for example: Everhart and Aust 2006). This argument is inadequate, if only because it is anthropocentric. The most-common form of violence globally, by far, is by humans towards animals for the production of food and so forth. This reality has rarely been depicted by WDAS even though animals are depicted in every WDAS film (1937–2016). Understood as violence (rather than as routine "food production processes"), no other form of violence comes remotely close in terms of the number of beings harmed. The number of animals slaughtered to produce food annually is higher than the number of all humans that die of any causes in a year, and that has been the case since the first WDAS film was released in 1937.[6] Yet, as this text has demonstrated, WDAS often attenuates, negates, or romanticizes the routine violence that animals face. For example, as Chap. 4 highlighted, Trusty the dog was supposed to die in the climax of *Lady and the Tramp*. However, this

[6] It is estimated that around three billion animals are killed every day (Zampa 2019). Since there are only an estimated 7.7 billion humans in the world, the amount of humans that die every day is undoubtedly far less than the number of animals killed (*World Population Review* 2019).

scene was changed after it was decided that such a moment would be too upsetting for children (Gavin 2015: 149, 480). WDAS also routinely attenuates violence towards animals where it occurs in a film's source text. This can be seen with *Dalmatians*, as was evidenced in Chap. 3. Therefore, where scenes are deemed to contain too much violence or harm towards animals, WDAS frequently attenuates, minimizes, and/or romanticizes it, so as to not upset audience sensibilities. As such, WDAS contributes to the cultural invisibility of such violence by downplaying the scale of harm done to animals. However, even though WDAS has mostly negated animal harm and objectification, they have commonly depicted the products of animal harm and objectification, such as meat, leather, and even locations in which animals are commonly harmed, such as farms and pet shops. Yet WDAS rarely depicts the processes by which animals are turned into objects. No WDAS film depicts a farm cow being slaughtered, yet several WDAS films feature cows as living characters, as well as other characters eating meat and wearing leather. This omission is important because visibility is needed to encourage a change in attitudes towards these practices.

Furthermore, this book has demonstrated that animal harm that is more visible to audiences in their everyday lived reality—such as those that can be incurred when animals are used for entertainment, kept as pets, or hunted—are less socially-acceptable than harms that are frequently occluded, such as those harms incurred during farming. Therefore, WDAS films reflect and propagate widespread reluctance to confront such harms. WDAS displays little interest in challenging the status quo wherein animals are harmed. However, WDAS clearly is interested in using animals, and the products created from their bodies, as central facets of their narratives, in order to create engaging stories that audiences want to watch. Therefore, contrary to those who suggest that WDAS films contain too much violence then, it is argued here that there is *not enough* violence in WDAS films. Moreover, by occluding the harm done to animals while simultaneously frequently depicting animals, WDAS films commit a symbolic harm towards animals. This is because the misleading depictions of animals in WDAS films can be detrimental towards the cause for better welfare. Again, visibility of these issues is necessary for change.

Approximately three billion animals are intentionally killed every day for human benefit (Zampa 2019). Most of these animals lead severely restricted lives and are physically harmed by their inadequate living conditions. Of these three billion deaths, many will be painful and violent. The lives and deaths of these nameless animals will go uncounted, undocumented, and will be quickly forgotten. In contrast, WDAS's cast of animal characters—found in films that centralise animals as lead protagonists (such as *Dumbo*), or films in which the entire cast are comprised of animals (such as *The Lion King*)—are remembered and treasured by audiences (for example: Clarke et al. 2017). Thus, WDAS films separate animals from their most common cause of death, which is the violence inflicted by humans.

As established at various points in this book, Walt was fond of animals. They inspired his most famous characters and works, such as Mickey Mouse, *Bambi*, *The Jungle Book*, and so forth. Therefore, Walt, WDAS, and Disney, owe their unique global success to animals. In a small way, WDAS does pay homage to animals, yet they have continuously ignored the harsh lives that most animals today experience. This text is of the opinion that all animals are sentient and can feel pain. However, given the reality and scale of animal harm today, one should hope that this position is incorrect. One should hope that WDAS is right; fish are objects, wild animals want to live in captivity, dogs desire human owners, cows are happy to lactate milk for other species, and so forth. Disney's depictions of animal harm are hopefully the ones that are correct because if animals do have lives of their own, away from the selfishness of humans, then companies like Disney have made a huge mistake.

Despite the frequently anthropomorphised depictions offered in WDAS films, non-human animals cannot speak for themselves. They cannot fight for the rights and laws that they need to protect them from the harms inflicted by humans. Animals are almost certainly incapable of understanding how they have been depicted in cultural representations, such as WDAS films. They cannot alter the attitudes humans have towards their species, which are developed and sustained through cultural depictions, such as WDAS films. Moreover, animals cannot understand the importance humans place on neoteny, anthropomorphism, individuality, and so forth. However, human judgements of an animal's "value" are shaped by those ideas. Furthermore, animals have no apparent interest in and cannot take pleasure from film in the same way that humans can. Cultural representations of animals can aid conservation and promote animal welfare. However, cultural representations can also perpetuate ideas about animals that are misleading, and they can entirely misrepresent the ways in which animals are routinely harmed by humans. At present, the latter kind of cultural presentation seems to far outweigh the former. As the harm-causing species and as the species with the most power in this dynamic, humans bear the responsibility to prevent harm to animals. Yet cultural representations of animals, such as WDAS films, have the power to impact the lives of billions of animals, so they should use these powers to do more.

Previous academic studies have helped to raise awareness about other forms of discrimination, and those interventions have helped to shift social and cultural attitudes more broadly. For example, the work of feminist scholars has raised consciousness about discriminatory depictions of women in the cultural sphere. When coupled with campaigning for legal changes to enshrine gender equality, that work helped to shift the baseline of normative attitudes. To illustrate, Davis (2015) suggests that WDAS stopped using female villains after much criticism that such characters were anti-feminist (2015: 244). Scholars concerned with speciesism can follow the same model to encourage changes in social attitudes towards animals. There is insufficient research into animal harm. This is a problem because research can lead to change. Animal harm and objectification are affecting animals, humans, and the environment in catastrophic ways. While WDAS films have received a generous amount of academic attention, animal harm and objectification have not received as much as they should have given the stakes: the routine harm inflicted upon billions of animals every day.

Appendixes

This data documents how many times each animal species is depicted in WDAS films (1937–2016). It also records how often animal harm and objectification (such as hunting) are depicted, along with locations (such as pet shops) in which animals are sometimes harmed. All fifty-six WDAS films (1937–2016) have been viewed five times each to record this information. This data impartially demonstrates how often WDAS has depicted animals, and the harms they experience. Therefore, it offers an objective history of how animals and animal harm have been depicted by WDAS, with no comment on these portrayals from the author of this book.

As with all data, there are some limitations to be noted. First, this data only documents and explores the harm and objectification experienced by extant non-human animal species. Extinct and mythical species are not being included in this data because these animals cannot face any harm or objectification in reality. Additionally, almost-all extinct and mythical animals are not based upon real species, so there is nothing to compare them with in reality. Second, in animated films, it is not always clear which species or object is being depicted. For example, as noted in Chapter 2, WDAS's representations of fish are often ambiguous; they are not based on any clear species of fish. Such characters lack detail and distinguishing features. These animals are counted within their respective species

R. R. Stanton, *The Disneyfication of Animals*, The Palgrave Macmillan Animal Ethics Series, https://doi.org/10.1007/978-3-030-49316-5

category as "ambiguous fish", "ambiguous birds", and so forth. Similarly, objectified animal-forms, such as leather, can also be ambiguous. The data recorded "leather" as any item that plausibly and contextually appeared to be leather, such as brown belts, black shoes, and so forth. However, it must be accepted the animators may not have been seeking to depict leather in such cases. Third, some species can only be defined by their wider taxonomic species category. For example, there are over 2000 known species of jellyfish (Gershwin 2016: 56). However, this book counts all species of jellyfish as jellyfish. This is again because specific species or breeds are not always clearly defined in animation. Fourth, animals that exist through metamorphosis are included in the data. For example, each species Melvin the wizard morphs into in *The Sword in the Stone* (1963) is included because they are identifiable. Fifth, hybrid animals (such as mermaids) are not included, even when based upon two extant species. This is because all of WDAS's hybrids are mythical hybrids, such as centaurs. WDAS has never depicted a real hybrid animal, such as a liger. Thus, as with the first limitation, there is no species to compare these characters to in reality. Sixth, ornaments, dolls, toys, and so forth based upon animals (such as teddy bears) are not included. Only living animals are included. For example, the animal-based ornaments in *Pinocchio* are not included. Seventh, still images of animals are also not being included in this text's data count. Only animals that move in some way are included. For example, in the opening of *Snow White*, a peacock is depicted in a book. However, this peacock is not included in this text's species count as it does not depict a moving animal. Eighth, only animated animals are being included in the film's data count. A small number of WDAS films, such as *Saludos Amigos* (1942) and *Fun and Fancy Free* (1947), contain live-action scenes. Any animals, harms, or instances of objectification in these scenes, such as the live-action donkeys in *Saludos Amigos*, are not included here. However, any animated animals in live-action scenes are included. For example, *The Three Caballeros* features several live-action scenes that include animated characters such as Donald Duck. The animated animals in those scenes are included here. Real animals are not being included as they cannot be interpreted in the same way that animated animals can be. Ninth, only animals that appear on screen visually are counted. For example, in *The Jungle Book*, frog ribbits are heard, yet frogs are not depicted on-screen. Therefore, frogs are not included in *The Jungle Book*'s count. Tenth, this book only studies intentional human-on-animal harm and objectification. For example, it does not include animal-on-animal hunting or animal-animal pet ownership. Moreover, it also does not include harms that are accidental. Eleventh, the species counted have been based upon the author's own perception of that species, which could occasionally be mistaken. Similarly, the author may be (unconsciously) biased towards certain species. Each film has been viewed five times to ensure that the results are as accurate as possible. Twelfth, all WDAS films were watched in their original, unedited, formats. Some scenes and characters have been removed from recent edits of WDAS films because they depict a person or situation that is no longer considered socially-acceptable. For example, this text's analysis of *Make Mine Music* (1946) includes "The Martin and the Coys", a segment that is almost-always removed from modern edits because of its comedic gunplay (Roberts 2018).

The species count conducted for this text is available at: https://rebeccarosestanton.wixsite.com/mysite. Because of the size of this data, it is not possible to include it neatly in this text.

Chapter 1: Animal Farming

Below is a list of all of the depictions of farm animals, farm locations, and the products of animal farming in WDAS films, presented in chronological order:

		Dairy	Eggs	Meat	Farm location	Chickens	Cows	Pigs
Snow White...	**1937**							
Pinocchio	**1940**	Y		Y				
Fantasia	**1940**							
Dumbo	**1941**			Y				
Bambi	**1942**							
Saludos Amigos	**1942**			Y			Y	
The Three...	**1944**					Y	Y	
Make Mine Music	**1946**	Y	Y		Y	Y		Y
Fun and Fancy...	**1947**	Y		Y	Y		Y	
Melody Time	**1948**		Y	Y	Y		Y	
The Adventures...	**1949**	Y	Y	Y	Y	Y	Y	Y
Cinderella	**1950**	Y				Y		
Alice in...	**1951**							

(continued)

(continued)

Peter Pan	**1953**							
Lady and....	**1955**			Y	Y	Y		
Sleeping Beauty	**1959**	Y	Y	Y				
101 Dalmatians	**1961**	Y		Y	Y		Y	
Sword in...	**1963**	Y		Y		Y		Y
The Jungle Book	**1967**							
The Aristocats	**1970**	Y		Y				
Robin Hood	**1973**					Y		Y
Winnie the Pooh	**1977**	Y						Y
The Rescuers	**1977**							
The Fox...	**1981**	Y			Y	Y	Y	
The Black...	**1985**			Y	Y			Y
The Great ...	**1986**	Y						
Oliver &...	**1988**	Y	Y	Y				
The Little...	**1989**	Y				Y		
The Rescuers...	**1990**		Y					
Beauty and...	**1991**	Y	Y	Y	Y	Y		Y
Aladdin	**1992**			Y		Y		
The Lion King	**1994**			Y				
Pocahontas	**1995**			Y	Y			
The Hunchback...	**1996**	Y		Y		Y		Y
Hercules	**1997**		Y	Y	Y	Y		
Mulan	**1998**		Y	Y	Y	Y	Y	Y
Tarzan	**1999**							
Fantasia 2000	**1999**	Y					Y	
Dinosaur	**2000**							
The Emperor's...	**2000**	Y		Y		Y	Y	Y
Atlantis: TLE	**2001**			Y				
Lilo & Stitch	**2002**	Y		Y				
Treasure Planet	**2002**							
Brother Bear	**2003**							
HOTR	**2004**	Y	Y	Y	Y	Y	Y	Y
Chicken Little	**2005**					Y	Y	Y
Meet the...	**2007**			Y			Y	
Bolt	**2008**			Y				
The Princess...	**2009**	Y	Y			Y	Y	Y
Tangled	**2010**			Y				
Winnie the Pooh	**2011**	Y						Y
Wreck-it Ralph	**2012**	Y	Y					
Frozen	**2013**	Y		Y				
Big Hero 6	**2014**			Y				
Zootopia	**2016**	Y					Y	Y
Moana	**2016**			Y	Y	Y		Y
		Dairy	**Eggs**	**Meat**	**Farm location**	**Chickens**	**Cows**	**Pigs**
	Totals	**25**	**12**	**30**	**14**	**19**	**15**	**16**
		45%	**21%**	**54%**	**25%**	**34%**	**27%**	**29%**

Chapter 2: Hunting and Fishing

Below are all of the instances of hunting and fishing in the fifty-six WDAS films included in this text. This only includes human-on-animal hunting and fishing. For example, Nala's attempt to hunt Pumba in *The Lion King* (1994) is not included as this is animal-on-animal hunting. Additionally, the live action fishing scenes in *Saludos Amigos* (1942) and *The Three Caballeros* (1942) are not included since they are live-action, not animated.

Pinocchio (1940)

Fishing: Slightly-anthropomorphised tuna fish are fished by Geppetto (a male human) with a fishing rod. It is implied that the fish die.

Bambi (1942)

Hunting: Deer, pheasants, and other forest wildlife are hunted by nameless human male hunters. The hunters use shotguns as weapons, and several animals are killed.

Make Mine Music (1946)

Hunting: The "Peter and the Wolf" short depicts a boy (Peter) hunting with a shotgun. Peter successfully captures the wolf, which is later tied up alive but is not shown dead.

Fishing: During "The Whale Who Wanted to Sing at the Met", Willie the whale is harpooned by male sailors and dies.[1]

One Hundred and One Dalmatians (1961)

Hunting: Dalmatian puppies are unsuccessfully hunted by Cruella, plus her hired hitmen, Jasper and Horace. They use various weapons. No puppies are killed.

The Sword in the Stone (1963)

Hunting: Sir Kay and Arthur (male humans) are shown unsuccessfully attempting to hunt a non-anthropomorphised deer with a bow and arrow.

[1] Whilst whales are mammals, the practice of killing them is referred to as both fishing and hunting. It is being labelled as fishing here as this scene takes place in the sea.

***The Fox and the Hound* (1981)**

Hunting: Amos (a male human) is shown hunting various species of animals (but mainly foxes) using a shotgun and trained hunting dogs. He is successful off-screen and unsuccessful on-screen.

***The Little Mermaid* (1989)**

Fishing: The male human sailors are seen catching hundreds of mostly non-anthropomorphised fish with large fishing nets.

***The Rescuers Down Under* (1990)**

Hunting: Percival McLeach sets traps to capture various Australian animals, some of which are endangered. He uses old-fashioned traps along with a shotgun. McLeach successfully captures many animals, but he does not successfully kill any on-screen. However, he boasts about the many animals he has killed off-screen.

***Beauty and the Beast* (1991)**

Hunting: Gaston and LeFou are shown successfully hunting and killing non-anthropomorphised geese with shotguns.

***Pocahontas* (1995)**

Fishing: Men are shown fishing with nomadic wooden spears.

Hunting: The male Native Americans have bow and arrows, which implies that they are hunting animals, although this is never shown. Additionally, John Smith (one of the settlers) is depicted preparing to kill a bear with a shotgun, but Pocahontas stops him.

***Mulan* (1998)**

Fishing: During their military training, the (mostly-male) soldiers are shown being taught to fish with their bare hands. Mulan (the only female) is at first unsuccessful at this task, whereas the males are successful. However, after she completes her training, she is successful.

***Tarzan* (1999)**

Hunting: Clayton and his henchmen are shown unsuccessfully hunting anthropomorphised gorillas with shotguns to take back to England.

Fantasia 2000 **(1999)**

Fishing: During the "Piano Concerto No. 2" segment, fishermen are seen catching hundreds of non-anthropomorphised fish with a fishing net. The fish are boxed-up and sold, so they certainly die.

Brother Bear **(2003)**

Hunting: The three brothers are shown hunting bears with spears.

Fishing: The three brothers are depicted fishing non-anthropomorphised fish with nets.

The Princess and the Frog **(2009)**

Hunting: Three male hunters chase the anthropomorphised frogs with various weapons, such as nets and clubs. Their hunt is unsuccessful.

Moana **(2016)**

Fishing: Groups of men on Moana's island fish daily with baskets. They are successful as fish are shown dead.

Combined Numbers

- Eleven films (20%) feature human-on-animal hunting. Out of the eleven times humans hunt, four instances (36%) result in the definite death of an animal (*Bambi*, *The Fox and the Hound*, *Beauty and the Beast*, and *Brother Bear*). 91% of WDAS's hunters are male. There is only one female hunter (Cruella De Vil), and she is unsuccessful.
- Eight films (14%) feature humans fishing. In 87% of films, the fishers are male. WDAS has only depicted a female fishing once (*Mulan*). Out of the eight times humans are depicted fishing, seven instances result in the definite death of fish (*Pocahontas* does not explicitly depict fish being caught).

Chapter 3: Clothing and Other Products Produced from Animals

Below are all of the depictions of fur, leather, feathers, and shells in the fifty-six WDAS films of this study:

		Feathers	Fur	Leather	Shells
Snow White...	1937	Y		Y	
Pinocchio	1940	Y	Y	Y	
Fantasia	1940	Y			Y
Dumbo	1941	Y	Y		
Bambi	1942				
Saludos Amigos	1942		Y	Y	
The Three Caballeros	1944	Y		Y	
Make Mine Music	1946	Y	Y	Y	
Fun and Fancy Free	1947	Y		Y	
Melody Time	1948	Y	Y	Y	
The Adventures of...	1949	Y	Y	Y	
Cinderella	1950	Y		Y	
Alice in Wonderland	1951	Y	Y	Y	
Peter Pan	1953	Y	Y	Y	Y
Lady and the Tramp	1955		Y		
Sleeping Beauty	1959	Y		Y	
101 Dalmatians	1961		Y	Y	
Sword in the Stone	1963	Y	Y	Y	
The Jungle Book	1967			Y	
The Aristocats	1970	Y	Y	Y	
Robin Hood	1973	Y	Y	Y	
Winnie the Pooh	1977			Y	
The Rescuers	1977	Y	Y	Y	
The Fox and the Hound	1981		Y	Y	
The Black Cauldron	1985	Y	Y	Y	
The Great Mouse...	1986	Y	Y	Y	
Oliver & Company	1988	Y	Y	Y	
The Little Mermaid	1989				Y
The Rescuers Down...	1990		Y	Y	
Beauty and the Beast	1991	Y	Y	Y	
Aladdin	1992	Y	Y		
The Lion King	1994				
Pocahontas	1995	Y	Y	Y	Y
The Hunchback...	1996	Y	Y	Y	
Hercules	1997	Y	Y	Y	
Mulan	1998	Y	Y	Y	
Tarzan	1999			Y	

(continued)

(continued)

Fantasia 2000	1999	Y	Y	Y	
Dinosaur	2000				
The Emperor's...	2000	Y	Y	Y	
Atlantis: TLE	2001	Y	Y	Y	
Lilo & Stitch	2002			Y	Y
Treasure Planet	2002			Y	Y
Brother Bear	2003	Y	Y	Y	
HOTR	2004	Y	Y	Y	
Chicken Little	2005			Y	
Meet the Robinsons	2007			Y	
Bolt	2008			Y	
The Princess and...	2009	Y	Y	Y	Y
Tangled	2010	Y	Y	Y	
Winnie the Pooh	2011			Y	
Wreck-it Ralph	2012	Y			
Frozen	2013	Y	Y	Y	
Big Hero 6	2014			Y	
Zootopia	2016			Y	
Moana	2016	Y		Y	Y
		Feathers	**Fur**	**Leather**	**Shells**
		36	**33**	**47**	**8**
		64%	**59%**	**84%**	**14%**

Chapter 4: Pets and Working Animals

Unlike the previous data presented, it is necessary to add clear guidelines as to how the terms "pet" and "working animal" are being defined. This is because both terms are more subjective than the harms referenced previously. While pets are often quite easy to identify, the boundaries occasionally blur and overlap with other types of character, such as best friends, sidekicks, henchmen, and so forth. This is particularly true of anthropomorphised animals because they often take on a human role alongside their animal role. Therefore, to make the data as consistent as possible, the following guidelines have been followed when identifying pets and working animals in WDAS films.

First, only animals that are the pet of a human character are included. For example, Timothy Q. Mouse (*Dumbo*) is not included here because he is an elephant's pet. Second, the pet has to live with the human character on their property. For example, while Snow White is followed through the forest by various woodland creatures, they do not live in her castle or the dwarfs' house with her. Thus, they are not her pets. Third, stray animals, or animals that reasonably appear to be stray, are not included here. For example, the dogs in "The Legend of Sleepy Hollow" from *The Adventures of Ichabod and Mr. Toad* do not appear to have owners, so they are not included here. The exception to this is stray animals that find homes within their narrative, such as Tramp (*Lady and the Tramp*) and Mittens (*Bolt*). Fourth, not all pets included here are domesticated animals. This is because not all WDAS films are set in the Anglo-American context. For example, in *Aladdin*, Aladdin has a pet monkey, and Jafar has a pet parrot. Fifth, as with the other chapters of this text, only extant, non-mythical, animal species will be included here. For example, Mushu (Mulan's red dragon) is not included here because he is based upon a mythical animal. Sixth, pets of no clear species are also not being included. For example, the small yellow bird in *Lady and the Tramp* is not detailed enough to represent any clear species, so it will not be included here. Seventh, the pets counted must fall into the traditional subservient pet role. For example, Terk from *Tarzan* is not Tarzan's pet; she is his best friend that he grows up alongside in the jungle.

This data will also count WDAS's working animals. Each animal character will only be counted once, as either a pet or working animal, even though some working animals could be reasonably be considered pets and vice versa. A working animal will be considered any animal that has a job which aids humans. For example, Copper from *The Fox and the Hound* is listed only as a working animal because his main purpose is to assist a human with hunting. It is necessary to separate pets from working animals because they differ greatly in terms of characterization and anthropomorphism, as well as the types of harm and discrimination they face. As with pets, only working animals that exist alongside a human character are included in this data.

This data is also noting the names, genders, and level of anthropomorphism (or lack thereof) of WDAS's pets and working animals. There are three levels of anthropomorphism noted: 1. non-anthropomorphised, 2. anthropomorphised but mute, and 3. heavily-anthropomorphised. "Non-anthropomorphised" refers to an animal character that lacks any human-like behaviour or appearance. In WDAS films, this usually refers to background animals. "Anthropomorphised but mute" refers to animal characters that are anthropomorphised but cannot speak. It is often the case that these characters understand English and respond through gesture, facial expression, and so forth. Two examples of this level of anthropomorphism are Lucifer (*Cinderella*) and Djali the goat (*The Hunchback of Notre Dame*). "Heavily-anthropomorphised" refers to a character that has many human traits and can speak English, such as Lady (*Lady and the Tramp*) or Pongo (*Dalmatians*).[2]

Snow White and the Seven Dwarves (1937)

Pets: Raven (genderless, nameless, villainous, anthropomorphised but mute).

Working animals: Horses for transport (genderless, nameless, non-anthropomorphised).

Deer for pulling loads (nameless, genderless, anthropomorphised but mute).

Pinocchio (1940)

Pets: Figaro the kitten (male, anthropomorphised but mute).

Cleo the goldfish (female, anthropomorphised but mute).

Working animals: Donkeys for pulling loads (genderless, nameless, non-anthropomorphised).

Bambi (1942)

Working animals: Dogs for hunting (genderless, nameless, non-anthropomorphised).

Saludos Amigos (1942)

Working animals: Llamas for carrying loads (genderless, nameless, anthropomorphised but mute).

---

[2] This may seem like a very simple way to categorize the complex anthropomorphism of WDAS's animal characters; however, this book is not about anthropomorphism, it is about the harms that animals experience. Therefore, the purpose of noting the level of anthropomorphism here is to compare how differently working animals and pets have been depicted. For this reason, this scale of anthropomorphism is adequate for the purpose of this text.

Horses for transport (genderless, nameless, anthropomorphised but mute).

***The Three Caballeros* (1944)**
Working animals: Horses for transport (genderless, nameless, anthropomorphised but mute).

***Make Mine Music* (1946)**
Working animals: Horses for transport (genderless, nameless, non-anthropomorphised).

***Fun and Fancy Free* (1947)**
Pets: Goldfish (female, nameless, anthropomorphised but mute).
Cat[3] (male, nameless, anthropomorphised but mute).

***Melody Time* (1948)**
Pets: Dogs (genderless, nameless, anthropomorphised but mute).
Cats (genderless, nameless, anthropomorphised but mute).
Working animals: Horses for transport (genderless, nameless, anthropomorphised but mute).
Cattle for pulling loads (genderless, nameless, non-anthropomorphised).

***The Adventures of Ichabod and Mr. Toad* (1949)**
Working animals: Police dogs (genderless, nameless, non-anthropomorphised).
Horses for transport (genderless, nameless, anthropomorphised but mute).

***Cinderella* (1950)**
Pets: Lucifer the cat (male, villainous, anthropomorphised but mute).
Bruno the dog (male, anthropomorphised but mute).
Working animals: Horses for transport (genderless, nameless, non-anthropomorphised).

[3] Jiminy Cricket refers to the cat as "son", implying that the cat is male.

***Alice in Wonderland* (1951)**

Pets: Dinah the cat (female, anthropomorphised but mute).

***Peter Pan* (1953)**

Pets: Nana the dog (female, anthropomorphised but mute).

***Lady and the Tramp* (1955)**

Pets: Pet dogs (mixed-gendered group, individually-named, heavily-anthropomorphised).

Si & Am the cats (female, villainous, heavily-anthropomorphised).

Yellow angel fish (genderless, nameless, anthropomorphised but mute).

This film also features a pet shop and a pound.

Working animals: Horses for transport (genderless, nameless, non-anthropomorphised).

***Sleeping Beauty* (1959)**

Pets: Diablo the raven (male, villainous, anthropomorphised but mute).

Working animals: Horses for transport (genderless, nameless, non-anthropomorphised). The one exception to this is Samson, Prince Phillip's anthropomorphised male horse.

***One Hundred and One Dalmatians* (1961)**[4]

Pets: Dogs (mixed-gendered group, individually-named, heavily-anthropomorphised).

This film also features a pet shop.

***The Sword in the Stone* (1963)**

Pets: Archimedes the owl (male, heavily-anthropomorphised).

Dogs (genderless, nameless, anthropomorphised but mute).

Working animals: Horses for transport (genderless, nameless, anthropomorphised but mute).

***The Aristocats* (1970)**

Pets: Cats (mixed-gendered group, individually-named, heavily-anthropomorphised).

---

[4] The horse-riding shown within the film that the puppies watch is not included here.

Working animals: Frou-Frou the horse for transport (female, heavily-anthropomorphised).

***The Rescuers* (1977)**

Pets: Brutus and Nero the crocodiles (male, villainous, anthropomorphised but mute).

Rufus the cat (male, heavily-anthropomorphised).

***The Fox and the Hound* (1981)**

Pets: Tod the fox (male, heavily-anthropomorphised).

Working animals: Chief and Copper, two hunting dogs (male, heavily-anthropomorphised).

***The Black Cauldron* (1985)[5]**

Pets: Cat (male, nameless, anthropomorphised but mute).

***The Great Mouse Detective* (1986)[6]**

Working animals: Horses for transport (genderless, nameless, non-anthropomorphised).

***Oliver & Company* (1988)**

Pets: Dogs (mixed-gendered group, individually-named, heavily-anthropomorphised).

Oliver the cat (male, heavily-anthropomorphised).

Goldfish (genderless, nameless, non-anthropomorphised).

Working animals: Roscoe and DoSoto for protection (male, heavily-anthropomorphised).

Horses for transport (genderless, nameless, non-anthropomorphised).

***The Little Mermaid* (1989)[7]**

Pets: Max the dog (male, anthropomorphised but mute).

Working animals: Horses for transport (genderless, nameless, non-anthropomorphised).

---

[5] Hen Wen the pig is not being included here as she is a farm animal. Additionally, the Horned King's guard dog is not included since the Horned King is not human.

[6] Most of this film features only animal characters. The data noted here refers to the large horse and cart depicted at the beginning of the film that is clearly transporting human characters.

[7] Ariel is being counted as a mermaid in this text. Thus, she is not human and her pets do not count.

The Rescuers down Under **(1990)**

Pets: Joanna the lizard (female, anthropomorphised but mute).

Beauty and the Beast **(1991)**

Working animals: Horses for transport (genderless, nameless, non-anthropomorphised). The exception to this is Belle's horse Philippe (male, anthropomorphised but mute).

Aladdin **(1992)**

Pets: Abu the monkey (male, anthropomorphised but mute).

Rajar the tiger (male, anthropomorphised but mute).

Iago the parrot (male, villainous, heavily-anthropomorphised).

Working animals: Camels for carrying loads (genderless, nameless, anthropomorphised but mute).

Horses for transport (genderless, nameless, anthropomorphised but mute).

Pocahontas **(1995)**

Pets: Meeko the raccoon (male, anthropomorphised but mute).

Flit the hummingbird (male, anthropomorphised but mute).

Percy the dog (male, villainous, anthropomorphised but mute).

Working animals: Horses for transport (genderless, nameless, non-anthropomorphised).

The Hunchback of Notre Dame **(1996)**

Pets: Djali the goat (male, anthropomorphised but mute).

Working animals: Horses for transport (genderless, nameless, non-anthropomorphised). Captain Phoebus also has an anthropomorphised (but mute) male horse called Achilles.

Hercules **(1997)**

Pets: Snowball the cat (genderless, anthropomorphised but mute).

Working animals: Horses for transport (genderless, nameless, non-anthropomorphised).

***Mulan* (1998)**

Pets: Hayabusa the falcon (male, villainous, anthropomorphised but mute).

Cri-kee the cricket (male, anthropomorphised but mute).

Little Brother the dog (male, anthropomorphised but mute).

Working animals: Horses for transport (genderless, nameless, non-anthropomorphised).

Cattle for transport (genderless, nameless, non-anthropomorphised).

Donkeys for transport (genderless, nameless, non-anthropomorphised).

***Fantasia 2000* (1999)**

Pets: Dog (genderless, nameless, non-anthropomorphised).

Working animals: Horses for transport (genderless, nameless, non-anthropomorphised).

"Rhapsody in Blue" also features a pet shop.

***The Emperor's New Groove* (2000)**

Working animals: Llamas for pulling loads (genderless, nameless, anthropomorphised but mute).

***Atlantis: The Lost Empire* (2001)**

Pets: Goldfish (genderless, nameless, non-anthropomorphised).

Fluffy the cat (genderless, anthropomorphised but mute).

Working animals: Horses for transport (genderless, nameless, non-anthropomorphised).

***Lilo and Stitch* (2002)**

This film features an animal pound/shelter.

***Brother Bear* (2003)**

Pets: Dog (genderless, nameless, non-anthropomorphised).

***Home on the Range* (2004)**

Working animals: Horses for transport (genderless, nameless, anthropomorphised but mute). Buck the horse (male, heavily-anthropomorphised).

Rusty the police dog (male, heavily-anthropomorphised).

***Meet the Robinsons* (2007)**

Pets: Buster the dog (male, non-anthropomorphised).

***Bolt* (2008)**

Pets: Bolt the dog (male, heavily-anthropomorphised).

Mittens the cat (female, heavily-anthropomorphised).

Rhino the hamster (male, heavily-anthropomorphised).

This film also features an animal shelter/pound.

***The Princess and the Frog* (2009)**

Pets: Stella the dog (female, anthropomorphised but mute).

Cat (genderless, nameless, anthropomorphised but mute).

Juju the snake (male, anthropomorphised but mute).

Working animals: Horses for transport (genderless, nameless, non-anthropomorphised).

***Tangled* (2010)**

Pets: Pascal the lizard (male, anthropomorphised, but mute).

Working animals: Horses for transport (genderless, nameless, non-anthropomorphised). The exception to this is Flynn's horse Maximus (male, anthropomorphised but mute).

***Frozen* (2013)**

Working animals: Horses for transport (genderless, nameless, non-anthropomorphised).

Reindeer for transport (genderless, nameless, non-anthropomorphised).

The two exceptions to this are Sitron the horse (male) and Sven the reindeer (male). Both are anthropomorphised but mute.

***Big Hero 6* (2014)**

Pets: Mochi the cat (genderless, anthropomorphised but mute).

***Moana* (2016)**

Pets: Hei Hei the chicken (male, anthropomorphised but mute)

Pua the pig (male, anthropomorphised but mute)

Combined Numbers[8]

- Animal shelters/pounds are featured in three films (5%).
- Pet shops are featured in three films (5%).
- Pets are featured in thirty-two films (57%). Across these thirty-two films, there are fifty-four different pets or same-species groups of pets.[9]
- Working animals are featured in thirty films (54%). Across these thirty films, there are forty different working animal characters or same-species groups of characters.[10]

WDAS's Pets

- Fifteen films feature cats as pets (27%). Fifteen films feature dogs as pets (27%). Four films feature goldfish as pets (7%). Two films feature lizards and ravens as pets (4%). Angel fish, chickens, crocodiles, crickets, falcons, foxes, goats, hamsters, hummingbirds, monkeys, owls, parrots, pigs, raccoons, snakes, and tigers, are each depicted in one film as a pet (2% each).
- Pets are mammals in thirty-seven films (69%). Birds are pets in seven films (13%). Fish are pets in five films (9%). Reptiles are pets in four films (7%). Insects are pets once (2%).
- In thirty-six cases (67%), pets are anthropomorphised but mute. In thirteen cases, pets are heavily-anthropomorphised (24%). In five instances, pets are not anthropomorphised at all (9%).
- Twenty-nine pets are male (54%), eight are female (15%), thirteen are without a clear gender (24%), and four exist in mixed-gender groups of their species (7%).

---

[8] The numbers have been rounded-up/down to one decimal place.

[9] Each species is being counted once per film. For example, even though *Lady and the Tramp* contains several pet dogs, dogs are only being counted once in this film. *Lady and the Tramp* contains three different species of pet (dog, cat, and fish), so this film has three pets. The data is being counted in this way to ensure that the results are not imbalanced.

[10] This is counted in the same way as with pets. Please see the previous footnote.

- Forty-one pets have names (76%), and thirteen are nameless (24%).
- Nine of WDAS's pets are villainous (17%).

Working Animals[11]

- Twenty-six films feature horses as working animals (65%). Five films feature dogs as working animals (12.5%). Two films feature donkeys, cattle, and/or llamas (5%). Camels, deer, and reindeer appear in one film each (2.5% each). Therefore, all of WDAS's working animals are mammals.
- In eleven films, working animals are anthropomorphised, but mute (27.5%). In twenty-five films, working animals are not anthropomorphised at all (62.5%). In four films, working animals are heavily anthropomorphised and can speak (10%).
- In thirty-six films, working animals are genderless (90%). In three films, they are male (7.5%). In one film, they are female (2.5%).
- The purposes of working animals are as follows: animals are used for riding/human transport in twenty-nine films (72.5%); animals are used for carrying goods in six films (15%); animals are used for animal hunting or as a police animal in two films each (5%); animals are used for protection in one film (2.5%).
- In thirty-six cases (90%), working animals are nameless. In four cases (10%), most of the working-animals have names.

[11] As noted in the data, some of the films feature many horses that are non-anthropomorphised, genderless, and nameless, but then they also have one horse that is named, gendered, and slightly-anthropomorphised. This is the case in *Sleeping Beauty*, *Beauty and the Beast*, and *The Hunchback of Notre Dame*, amongst others. In these cases, the data counts what is the norm for the majority of working animals in that film. For example, in *Sleeping Beauty*, there is one anthropomorphised horse and hundreds of non-anthropomorphised horses. Therefore, this data counts the horses in *Sleeping Beauty* as non-anthropomorphised, nameless, and genderless, as that is the case for almost-all horses in that film. In contrast, in some films, all, or almost all, of the working animals are individualized. For example, in *The Fox and the Hound*, the two hunting dogs have names, genders, and so forth. In these instances, the working animals are counted as heavily-anthropomorphised, gendered, and so forth as this is the norm for working animals in that film.

Bibliography

About Britain (2009–2019) *Britain's best zoos.* Available at: https://about-britain.com/tourism/zoos-wildlife.htm (Accessed: 4 July 2019).

Adams, C. J. (2010) *The Sexual Politics of Meat: a Feminist-Vegetarian Critical Theory 20th anniversary edition.* London: Continuum.

Adams, S. (2009) 'Karl Lagerfeld Defends Fur Industry Saying 'Beasts' Would Kill Us if We Didn't Kill Them', *The Telegraph*, 2 January. Available at: http://fashion.telegraph.co.uk/news-features/TMG4075783/Karl-Lagerfeld-defends-fur-industry-saying-beasts-would-kill-us-if-we-didnt-kill-them.html (Accessed: 23 June 2018).

AFI: American Film Institute Catalog of Motion Pictures Produced in the United States: Feature Films, 1941–1950 (1999). Berkeley: University of California Press.

Agerholm, H. (2018) 'Hundreds of illegal hunts took place in British countryside last autumn, animal rights group says', *Independent*, 3 April. Available at: https://www.independent.co.uk/news/uk/home-news/hunts-illegal-hundreds-autumn-season-figures-animal-rights-hunting-ban-england-wales-a8286336.html (Accessed: 4 December 2018).

Aldrich, B. C. (2018) 'The Use of Primate "Actors" in Feature Films 1990–2013', *Anthrozoös*, 31(1), pp. 5–21.

R. R. Stanton, *The Disneyfication of Animals*, The Palgrave Macmillan Animal Ethics Series, https://doi.org/10.1007/978-3-030-49316-5

American Film Institute (2017) *Lady and the Tramp*. Available at: https://catalog.afi.com/Catalog/moviedetails/51552 (Accessed: 8 July 2019).

American Film Institute (2019) *AFI's 100 Greatest Heroes & Villains*. Available at: https://www.afi.com/100years/handv.aspx (Accessed: 13 June 2019).

American Humane (2019a) *About Us*. Available at: https://www.americanhumane.org/about-us/ (Accessed: 26 March 2019).

American Humane (2019b) *Governance*. Available at: https://www.americanhumane.org/about-us/governance-and-finances/ (Accessed: 7 May 2019).

American Humane (2019c) *Guidelines for the Safe Use of Animals in Filmed Media*. Available at: https://www.americanhumane.org/app/uploads/2016/08/Guidelines2015-WEB-Revised-110315-1.pdf (Accessed: 28 April 2019).

American Humane (2019d) *History*. Available at: https://www.americanhumane.org/about-us/history/ (Accessed: 7 April 2019).

American Humane (2019e) *Independent Investigative Report on "A Dog's Purpose" Finds Edited Video Mischaracterized What Happened on the Set*. Available at: https://www.americanhumane.org/press-release/independent-investigative-report-on-a-dogs-purpose-finds-edited-video-mischaracterized-what-happened-on-the-set/ (Accessed: 12 March 2019).

American Humane (2019f) *"No Animals Were Harmed" We Help Keep the Cameras Rolling and the Animals Safe*. Available at: https://www.americanhumane.org/initiative/no-animals-were-harmed/ (Accessed: 7 May 2019).

Anderson, M. V. and Henderson, A. J. Z. (2005) 'Pernicious Portrayals: The Impact of Children's Attachment to Animals of Fiction on Animals of Fact', *Society and Animals*, 13(4), pp. 297–314.

Animal Equality (2019) *Entertainment*. Available at: https://www.animalequality.net/entertainment (Accessed: 4 June 2019).

Animation Source (2018) *Hmm… Something Looks Familiar*. Available at: https://www.animationsource.org/lady_tramp/en/articles/Hmm...-Something-Looks-Familiar/136001.html&id_film=25 (Accessed: 12 November 2018).

Arluke, A. and Sanders, C. R. (1996) *Regarding Animals*. Philadelphia: Temple University Press.

Arluke, A. (2006) *Just a Dog: Understanding Animal Cruelty and Ourselves*. Philadelphia: Temple University Press.

Artz, L. (2004) 'The Righteousness of Self-Centred Royals: The World According to Disney Animation', *Critical Arts*, 18(1), pp. 116–146.

ASPCA (2018) *About Us*. Available at: https://www.aspca.org/about-us (Accessed: 4 December 2018)

Assistance Dogs (2019) *Assistance Dogs UK*. Available at: http://www.assistance-dogs.org.uk/ (Accessed: 8 July 2019).

Atkins-Sayre, W. (2010) 'Articulating Identity: People for the Ethical Treatment of Animals and the Animal/Human Divide', *Western Journal of Communication*, 74(3), pp. 309–328.

Barnes, H. (2016) 'Watership Down Too Violent for Tots? Probably, but Parents Should Take Control of the Remote', *The Guardian*, 31 March. Available at: https://www.theguardian.com/film/filmblog/2016/mar/31/watership-down-bbfc-ratings-easter-sunday-comment (Accessed: 22 February 2019).

Barnett, A. (2006) 'The slaughtered horses that shame our racing', *The Guardian*, 1 October. Available at: https://www.theguardian.com/uk/2006/oct/01/horseracing.sport (Accessed: 22 February 2019).

Baron, K. (2016) 'Fashion's Greatest Pop Hits – from Gaga's Meat Dress to Grace Jones's Armani Suit', *The Guardian*, 16 August. Available at: https://www.theguardian.com/fashion/2016/aug/16/fashions-greatest-pop-hits-from-gagas-meat-dress-to-grace-joness-armani-suit (Accessed: 11 June 2019)

Barrier, M. J. (2007) *The Animated Man: A Life of Walt Disney*. Berkeley: University of California Press.

Barrier, M. (2011) *The Mysterious Dumbo Roll-A-Book*. Available at: http://www.michaelbarrier.com/Essays/DumboRollABook/DumboRollABook.html (Accessed: 15 February 2019).

Batt, S. (2009) 'Human attitudes towards animals in relation to species similarity to humans: a multivariate approach', *Bioscience Horizons: The International Journal of Student Research*, 2(1), pp. 180–190.

Baum, G. (2013a) 'Animals Were Harmed', *The Hollywood Reporter*, 25 November. Available at: https://www.hollywoodreporter.com/news/animals-were-harmed-hollywood-reporter-investigation-on-set-injury-death-cover-ups-659556 (Accessed: 15 September 2018).

Baum, G. (2013b) ''Life of Pi' AHA Monitor Leaves Job After THR Email Exposes Tiger 'Damn Near Drowned'', *The Hollywood Reporter*, 26 November. Available at: https://www.hollywoodreporter.com/news/life-pi-aha-monitor-leaves-660369 (Accessed: 15 September 2018).

BBC News (2017) *A Dog's Purpose Premiere Cancelled Amid Animal Rights Concerns*. Available at: https://www.bbc.com/news/world-us-canada-38695074 (Accessed: 23 December 2018).

BBFC (2010) *What Are You Complaining About Now?* Available at: https://www.bbfc.co.uk/education-resources/education-news/what-are-you-complaining-about-now (Accessed: 9 November 2018).

Beatson, R. M. and Halloran, M. J. (2010) 'Humans rule! The effects of creatureliness reminders, mortality salience and self-esteem on attitudes towards animals', *British Journal of Social Psychology*, 46(3), pp. 619–632.

Beck, J. (2005) *The Animated Movie Guide*. Chicago: Chicago Review Press.

Beiman, N. (2007) *Prepare to Board!: Creating Story and Characters for Animated Features and Shorts*. London: Taylor & Francis.

Beinart, P. (1995) 'The Fur Flies: an Activist's Nightmare. (Conflicts between Animal-Rights Activists and Indigenous Peoples)', *The New Republic*, 213(25), p. 11.

Bekhechi, M. (2010) 'Peta's persistence is opening people's eyes', *The Guardian*, 3 November. Available at: https://www.theguardian.com/commentisfree/cifamerica/2010/nov/03/peta-cruelty-to-animals (Accessed: 10 June 2017).

Bekoff, M. (2018) 'Cecil the Lion: His Life, Death, and Effects on Conservation An interview with Andrew Loveridge, author of Lion Hearted, who knew Cecil well', *Psychology Today*, 27 March. Available at: https://www.psychologytoday.com/us/blog/animal-emotions/201803/cecil-the-lion-his-life-death-and-effects-conservation (Accessed: 12 December 2018).

Bernard, M. (2011) 'Cannibalism, Class and Power: A Foodways Analysis of The Texas Chain Saw Massacre Series', *Food, Culture & Society*, 14(3), pp. 413–432.

Bettany, S. and Belk, R. W. (2011) 'Disney Discourses of Self and Other: Animality, Primitivity, Modernity, and Postmodernity', *Consumption Markets & Culture*, 14(2), pp. 163–176.

Betts, H. (2012) 'Why I'm Happy to Wear Fur', *The Guardian*, 18 September. Available at: https://www.theguardian.com/commentisfree/2012/sep/18/happy-wear-fur-vegetarian (Accessed: 3 March 2017).

BHWT (2019) *Beak Trimming: Mutilation or Necessary?* Available at: https://www.bhwt.org.uk/egg-industry/facts-beak-trimming/ (Accessed: 10 November 2018).

Black, R. (2011) 'Species Count Put at 8.7 Million', *BBC News*, 23 August. Available at: https://www.bbc.co.uk/news/science-environment-14616161 (Accessed: 28 June 2019).

Blue Cross (2019) *The Field Kept Horse*. Available at: https://www.bluecross.org.uk/pet-advice/field-kept-horse (Accessed: 8 July 2019).

Borgi, M. and Cirulli, F. (2015) 'Attitudes toward Animals among Kindergarten Children: Species Preferences', *Anthrozoös*, 28(1), pp. 45–59.

Borgi, M., and Cirulli, F. (2016) 'Pet Face: Mechanisms Underlying Human-Animal Relationships', *Frontiers in Psychology*, 7(298), pp. 1–11.

Borkfelt, S. (2011) 'What's in a Name? – Consequences of Naming Non-Human Animals', *Animals*, 1(1), pp. 116–125.

Born Free Foundation (2016) *The Use of Wild Animals in Performance 2016*. Available at: https://www.bornfree.org.uk/storage/media/content/files/Publications/PERFORMING_ANIMALS_REPORT_2016.pdf (Accessed: 5 March 2019).

Bowers, D. B. (2014) 'The Saga of Davy Crockett's Coonskin Cap', *American History*, 17 November. Available at: https://americanhistory.si.edu/blog/saga-davy-crocketts-coonskin-cap (Accessed: 5 May 2017).

Bowman, S. L. (2011) 'The Dichotomy of the Great Mother Archetype in Disney Heroines and Villainesses', in Heit, J. (ed.) *Vader, Voldemort, and other Villains: Essays on Evil in Popular Media*. Jefferson: McFarland & Company, pp. 80–96.

Box Office Mojo (2019) *Home on the Range*. Available at: https://www.boxofficemojo.com/movies/?id=homeontherange.htm (Accessed: 1 July 2019).

Boydell, R. (2016) 'The secret Daenerys wears under every dress: secrets from the Game Of Thrones costume director', *The Telegraph*, 25 April. Available at: https://www.telegraph.co.uk/fashion/people/the-secret-daenerys-wears-under-every-dress-secrets-from-the-gam/ (Accessed: 6 January 2019).

Brahic, C. (2009) 'Why freeing Willy was the wrong thing to do', *New Scientist*, 28 April. Available at: https://www.newscientist.com/article/dn17039-why-freeing-willy-was-the-wrong-thing-to-do/ (Accessed: 12 March 2019).

Bristol Zoo Gardens (2019) *Gorillas*. Available at: https://www.bristolzoo.org.uk/explore-the-zoo/ (Accessed: 4 July 2019).

Brooke, B. (2001) 'Step Right Up!', *History Magazine*, October/November issue. Available at: https://www.history-magazine.com/circuses.html (Accessed: 15 April 2019)

Brooks, X. (2012) 'Award Posthumous Oscar to dog star Rin Tin Tin, says biographer', *The Guardian*, 4 January. Available at: https://www.theguardian.com/film/2012/jan/04/award-oscar-dog-rin-tin-tin (Accessed: 17 April 2019).

Brown, C. (2015) 'Fish intelligence, sentience and ethics', *Animal Cognition*, 18(1), pp. 1–17.

Brown, D. (2001a) 'Phoenix, the calf they couldn't cull, fights on', *The Telegraph*, 25 April. Available at: https://www.telegraph.co.uk/news/uknews/1317136/Phoenix-the-calf-they-couldnt-cull-fights-on.html (Accessed: 25 July 2019).

Brown, P. (2001b) 'Last Mink Fur Farms Must Close by 2003', *The Guardian*, 28 December. Available at: https://www.theguardian.com/uk/2001/dec/28/immigrationpolicy (Accessed: 30 March 2017).

Brown, S. (2011) 'Do They Not Bleed? Industrial Agriculture and the Cruel Fate of Farm Animals', *Canadian Dimension*, 45(4), p. 23.

Browne, A. (2001) 'Calf? I nearly died', *The Guardian*, 29 April. Available at: https://www.theguardian.com/news/2001/apr/29/politics.footandmouth (Accessed: 28 February 2019).

Brucculieri, J. (2017) 'Josh Gad Responds to 'Disturbing' Leaked Video from 'A Dog's Purpose' Set [UPDATE]', *The Huffington Post*, 19 January. Available at: https://www.huffingtonpost.com/entry/josh-gad-a-dogs-purpose-video-response_us_5880be0ae4b04b69667e9e09 (Accessed: 4 January 2019).

Buller, H. (2013) 'Individuation, the Mass and Farm Animals', *Theory, Culture & Society*, 30(7–8), pp. 155–175.

Burt, J. (2002) *Animals in Film*. London: Reaktion Books.

Cameron, C. D., Payne, B. K., and Judd, C. M. (2011) 'Escaping Affect: How Motivated Emotion Regulation Creates Insensitivity to Mass Suffering', *Journal of Personality and Social Psychology*, 100(1), pp. 1–15.

Carter, C. (2014) 'Lassie and 101 Dalmatians influence popularity of dog breeds for up to ten years', *The Telegraph*, 10 September. Available at: https://www.telegraph.co.uk/lifestyle/pets/11086650/Lassie-and-101-Dalmatians-influence-popularity-of-dog-breeds-for-up-to-ten-years.html (Accessed: 14 September 2018).

Cartmill, M. (1996) *A View to a Death in the Morning: Hunting and Nature through History*. Cambridge: Harvard University Press.

Cataldi, S. L. (2002) 'Animals and the Concept of Dignity: Critical Reflections on a Circus Performance', *Ethics & the Environment*, 7(2), pp. 104–126.

Cave, J. (2017) 'Remembering Tyke, Rebellious Circus Elephant, And Her Tragic Death (GRAPHIC VIDEO)', *Huffington Post*, 19 August. Available at: https://www.huffpost.com/entry/tyke-elephant-honolulu-circus_n_5689932 (Accessed: 27 February 2019)

Cheu, J. (2013) *Diversity in Disney Films*. Jefferson: McFarland & Company.

Child, B. (2013) 'Life of Pi Tiger Nearly Drowned on Set, Report Alleges', *The Guardian*, 27 November. Available at: https://www.theguardian.com/film/2013/nov/27/life-of-pi-tiger-nearly-drowned-report-animals-hollywood (Accessed: 2 March 2018).

Choi, C. Q. (2010) 'How 'Jaws' Forever Changed Our View of Great White Sharks', *Live Science*, 10 June. Available at: https://www.livescience.com/8309-jaws-changed-view-great-white-sharks.html (Accessed: 26 August 2017).

Clarke, C., Rothkopf, J., Calhoun, D., Huddleston, T., and Uhlich, K. (2017) 'The best and worst Disney movies', *Time Out*, 30 March. Available at: https://www.timeout.com/london/film/disney-movies-list (Accessed: 22 February 2019).

Cochrane, E. (2014) '101 Dalmatians Review', *Empire*, 1 January. Available at: http://www.empireonline.com/movies/101-dalmatians/review/ (Accessed: 25 March 2018).

Cole, M. and Morgan, K. (2011) 'Vegaphobia: Derogatory Discourses of Veganism and the Reproduction of Speciesism in UK National Newspapers', *The British Journal of Sociology*, 62(1), pp. 134–153.

Cole, M. and Stewart, K. (2014) *Our Children and Other Animals: The Cultural Construction of Human-Animal Relations in Childhood*. Farnham: Ashgate Publishing.

Coleman, J. T. (2015) 'The Shoemaker's Circus: Grizzly Adams and Nineteenth-Century Animal Entertainment', *Environmental History*, 20(4), pp. 593–618.

Collin, R. (2017) 'The sad, strange saga of Independence Day hero Randy Quaid', *The Telegraph*, 4 July. Available at: https://www.telegraph.co.uk/films/2016/06/24/the-sad-strange-saga-of-independence-day-hero-randy-quaid/ (Accessed: 13 January 2019).

Connell, J. (2018) "Cows carry flesh, but they carry personality too': the hard lessons of farming', *The Guardian*, 22 March. Available at: https://www.theguardian.com/news/2018/mar/22/cows-carry-flesh-but-they-carry-personality-too-the-hard-lessons-of-farming (Accessed: 25 January 2019).

Cottee, S. Y. (2012) 'Are Fish the Victims of 'Speciesism'? A Discussion about Fear, Pain and Animal Consciousness', *Fish Physiology and Biochemistry*, 38(1), pp. 5–15.

Cummins, J. (1995). 'Romancing the Plot: The Real Beast of Disney's Beauty and the Beast', *Children's Literature Association Quarterly*, 20(1), pp. 22–28.

Dalton, J. (2019) 'Do companies still test toiletries and household cleaners on animals and how can you tell?' Independent, 23 April. Available at: https://www.independent.co.uk/infact/animal-testing-cruelty-free-cosmetics-toiletries-household-products-a8877221.html (Accessed: 22 September 2019).

David, S. (2018) 'America's Horrifying New Plan for Animals: Highspeed Slaughterhouses', *The Guardian*, 6 March. Available at: https://www.theguardian.com/commentisfree/2018/mar/06/ive-seen-the-hidden-horrors-of-high-speed-slaughterhouses (Accessed: 22 December 2018).

Davies, M. (2010) *Children, Media and Culture*. Maidenhead: McGraw-Hill Education.

Davis, A. M. (2007) *Good Girls and Wicked Witches*. Barnet: John Libbey.

Davis, A. M. (2015) *Handsome Heroes and Vile Villains: Masculinity in Disney's Feature Films*. Bloomington: Indiana University Press.

Davis, J. M. (2017) '"Pain Is the Only School-Teacher": the Jack London Club and the Politics of American Animal Performance, 1880–1945', *Early Popular Visual Culture*, 15(3), pp. 334–349.

Dearden, L. (2014) 'Simba, Bambi and other Disney characters shown skinned and bleeding in anti-fur campaign', *Independent*, 1 December. Available at: https://www.independent.co.uk/arts-entertainment/art/news/simba-bambi-and-disney-characters-shown-skinned-and-bleeding-in-anti-fur-campaign-9896355.html (Accessed: 16 March 2018).

Debenhams (2019) *Leather*. Available at: https://www.debenhams.com/gifts/leather-1 (Accessed: 27 July 2019).

Deckers, J. (2016) *Animal (De)Liberation: Should the Consumption of Animal Products Be Banned?* London: Ubiquity Press.

Deja, A. (2015) *The Nine Old Men: Lessons, Techniques, and Inspiration from Disney's Great Animators*. London: Routledge.

Diamond, W. (2017) 'Animals and the Academy Awards: A History', *Huffington Post*, 6 December. Available at: https://www.huffingtonpost.com/wendy-diamond/animals-and-the-academy-a_b_481290.html (Accessed: 22 November 2018).

Disneyland Paris (2019) *Disney's Davy Crockett Ranch*. Available at: https://www.disneylandparis.com/en-gb/hotels/disneys-davy-crockett-ranch/ (Accessed: 7 March 2019).

Disney World (2019) *Rooms & Packages – Frequently Asked Questions*. Available at: https://disneyworld.disney.go.com/en_GB/faq/rooms-packages/hotels-pet-friendly/ (Accessed: 1 April 2019).

Dobson, N. (2010) *The A-Z of Animation and Cartoons*. Lanham: Rowman & Littlefield.

Dockterman, E. and Conniff, K. (2014) 'Maleficent and 16 Other Famous Queens of Mean', *Time*, 31 May. Available at: http://time.com/2801704/maleficent-villains-wicked-witch-catwoman/ (Accessed: 2 June 2018).

Dodd, V. (2018) '"Croydon cat killer" hunt ends after three-year investigation', *The Guardian*, 20 September. Available at: https://www.theguardian.com/world/2018/sep/20/croydon-cat-killer-unmasked-after-three-year-investigation (Accessed: 11 December 2018).

Dogs Trust (2018) *Dogs Trust: A Dog is for Life, Not Just for Christmas*. Available at: https://www.dogstrust.org.uk/news-events/news/dogs-trust-a-dog-is-for-life-not-just-for-christmas (Accessed: 22 May 2019).

Donnelly, T. (2015) 'Why 'Jaws' terrifies even phobia experts', *New York Post*, 18 June. Available at: https://nypost.com/2015/06/18/why-jaws-terrifies-even-phobia-experts/ (Accessed: 12 January 2019).

Dorré, G. M. (2002) 'Horses and Corsets: "Black Beauty," Dress Reform, and the Fashioning of the Victorian Woman', *Victorian Literature and Culture*, 30(1), pp. 157–78.

Duffy, R. (2010) *Nature Crime: How We're Getting Conservation Wrong*. New Haven: Yale University Press.

Elder, M. P. (2014) 'The Fish Pain Debate: Broadening Humanity's Moral Horizon', *Journal of Animal Ethics*, 4(2), pp. 16–29.

Endenburg, N. and Vorstenbosch, J. M. G. (1992) 'Ethical issues in the ownership of companion animals: An empirical and normative analysis', *Veterinary Quarterly*, 14(4), pp. 129–136.

Estren, M. J. (2012) 'The Neoteny Barrier: Seeking Respect for the Non-Cute', *Journal of Animal Ethics*, 2(1), pp. 6–11.

Everhart, K. and Aust, P. J. (2006) 'What is your Child Watching? A Content Analysis of Violence in Disney Animated Films', *Kentucky Journal of Communication*, 25(2), pp. 101–127.

Fagan, B. (2018) *Fishing: How the Sea Fed Civilization*. New Haven: Yale University Press.

Farm Sanctuary (2018) *Wool, Leather, and Down*. Available at: https://www.farmsanctuary.org/learn/factory-farming/wool-leather-and-down/ (Accessed: 11 November 2018).

Fitzgerald, A. J., Kalof, L., and Dietz, T. (2009) 'Slaughterhouses and Increased Crime Rates: An Empirical Analysis of the Spillover From "The Jungle" Into the Surrounding Community', *Organization & Environment*, 22(2), pp. 158–184.

Fleming, P. C. (2016) 'Dickens, Disney, Oliver, and Company: Adaptation in a Corporate Media Age', *Children's Literature Association Quarterly*, 41(2), pp. 182–198.

Flynn, C. P. (2012) *Understanding Animal Abuse: A Sociological Analysis*. New York: Lantern Books.

Forbes, D. A. (2011) 'The Aesthetic of Evil', in Heit, J. (ed.) *Vader, Voldemort, and other Villains: Essays on Evil in Popular Media*. Jefferson: McFarland & Company, pp. 13–27.

Frammalino, R. and Bates, J. (2001) 'Questions Raised About Group That Watches Out for Animals in Movies', *Los Angeles Times*, 9 February. Available at: http://articles.latimes.com/2001/feb/09/news/mn-23161/3 (Accessed: 2 March 2019).

Freeman, C. P. (2009) 'This Little Piggy Went to Press: The American News Media's Construction of Animals in Agriculture', *The Communication Review*, 12(1), pp. 78–103.

Fur Free Alliance (2018) *Fur Farming*. Available at: https://www.furfreealliance.com/fur-farming/ (Accessed: 13 May 2018).

Garner, C. (1996) 'Film may cause 1001 unwanted Dalmatians', *The Independent*, 1 December. Available at: https://www.independent.co.uk/news/film-may-cause-1001-unwanted-dalmatians-1312437.html (Accessed: 16 March 2019).

Gartler, J. (2015) 'In Recognition of a Renaissance Man', *Animation World Network*, 23 March. Available at: https://www.awn.com/animationworld/recognition-renaissance-man (Accessed: 5 March 2019).

Gavin, J. (2015) *Is That All There Is?: The Strange Life of Peggy Lee*. New York: Simon & Schuster.

Gershwin, L. (2016) *Jellyfish: A Natural History*. Chicago: University of Chicago Press.

Ghirlanda S., Acerbi A., and Herzog, H. (2014) 'Dog Movie Stars and Dog Breed Popularity: A Case Study in Media Influence on Choice', in *PLOS ONE*, 9(9): e106565. https://doi.org/10.1371/journal.pone.0106565.

Golding, W. (1954) *Lords of the Flies: A Novel*. London: Faber & Faber.

Goldman, J. G. (2016) 'Why did the death of Cecil the lion cause such an uproar?', *The Guardian*, 5 May. Available at: https://www.theguardian.com/environment/2016/may/05/why-did-death-of-a-single-lion-cecil-cause-such-an-uproar (Accessed: 22 November 2018).

Goldmark, D. and McKnight, U. (2008) 'Locating America: Revisiting Disney's Lady and the Tramp', *Social Identities*, 14(1), pp. 101–120.

Gould, S. J. (1977) *Ontogeny and phylogeny*. Cambridge: Harvard University.

Gray, E. A. (2014) *Corporate Responsibility, Ethics, and Animal Welfare*. Master's Thesis. St Catherine University. Available at: https://sophia.stkate.edu/cgi/viewcontent.cgi?article=1029&context=maol_theses (Accessed: 11 June 2019).

Gray, J. (2017) *Zoo Ethics: The Challenges of Compassionate Conservation*. Ithaca: Cornell University Press.

Groneman, W. (2007) *David Crockett: Hero of the Common Man*. Forge Books.

Guide Dogs (2019) *About Us*. Available at: https://www.guidedogs.org.uk/about-us/ (Accessed: 8 July 2019).

Gunasekera, C. A. (2018) 'The Ethics of Killing "Surplus" Zoo Animals', *Journal of Animal Ethics*, 8(1), pp. 93–102.

Hadley, M. (2009) *Michael Jackson Master of Illusion: The Final Curtain Call.* Indiana: Xlibris.

Hance, J. (2016) 'Cecil's legacy: could the death of one lion start a conservation movement?', *The Guardian*, 27 April. Available at: https://www.theguardian.com/environment/radical-conservation/2016/apr/27/cecils-legacy-could-the-death-of-one-lion-start-a-conservation-movement (Accessed: 23 November 2018).

Hancox, D. (2018) 'The unstoppable rise of veganism: how a fringe movement went mainstream', *The Guardian*, 1 April. Available at: https://www.theguardian.com/lifeandstyle/2018/apr/01/vegans-are-coming-millennials-health-climate-change-animal-welfare (Accessed: 13 December 2018).

Harrods (2018) *Fur Coats*. Available at: https://www.harrods.com/en-gb/women/clothing/coats/fur-coats (Accessed: 12 April 2019).

Hastings, A. W. (1996) 'Bambi and the Hunting Ethos', *Journal of Popular Film and Television*, 24(2), pp. 53–59.

Hawkes, R. (2016) 'Remembering The Artist's Uggie: One of Cinema's Top Dogs', *The Telegraph*, 25 December. Available at: https://www.telegraph.co.uk/films/0/remembering-uggie-dog-star-artist-one-cinemas-charismatic-canines/ (Accessed: 4 March 2019).

Heching, D. (2020) 'Lady Gaga looks ready to rock and roll in black motorcycle leather jacket as she heads to the studio', The Daily Mail, 11 February. Available at: https://www.dailymail.co.uk/tvshowbiz/article-7993137/Lady-Gaga-looks-ready-rock-roll-black-motorcycle-leather-jacket.html (Accessed: 19 February 2020).

Henderson, A. and Anderson, M. (2005) 'Pernicious Portrayals: The Impact of Children's Attachment to Animals of Fiction on Animals of Fact', *Society & Animals*, 13(4), pp. 297–314.

Hill, S. and Broom, D. (2009) 'Measuring zoo animal welfare: Theory and practice', *Zoo Biology*, 28(6), pp. 531–44.

Hoad, P. (2014) 'Watership Down: the film that frightened me the most', *The Guardian*, 30 October. Available at: https://www.theguardian.com/film/filmblog/2014/oct/30/watership-down-the-film-that-frightened-me-the-most (Accessed: 2 February 2019).

Hoffman, M. and Ackerman, L. J. (1998) *Dogs: The Ultimate Care Guide: Good Health, Loving Care, Maximum Longevity*. London: Rodale Books.

Hollander, J. M. (2003) *The Real Environmental Crisis: Why Poverty, Not Affluence, Is the Environment's Number One Enemy*. Los Angeles: University of California Press.

Horta, O. (2010) 'What is Speciesism?', *Journal of Agricultural and Environmental Ethics*, 23(3), pp. 243–266.

Hribal, J. (2003) 'Animals are part of the working class": a challenge to labor history', *Labor History*, 44(4), pp. 435–453.

Humane Hollywood (2018a) *About the Film and Television Unit: No Animals Were Harmed*. Available at: http://humanehollywood.org/index.php/component/content/article/10-reviews/30-about-the-film-television-unit (Accessed: 7 September 2018).

Humane Hollywood (2018b) *A Long History of Ensuring Safety*. Available at: http://www.humanehollywood.org/index.php/end-credits/end-credit-evolution (Accessed: 11 September 2018).

Humane Hollywood (2018c) *Certification Definition*. Available at: http://humanehollywood.org/index.php/on-the-set/certification-definition (Accessed: 7 September 2018).

Humane Hollywood (2018d) *Eight Below*. Available at: http://humanehollywood.org/index.php/movie-archive/item/eight-below (Accessed: 11 September 2018).

Humane Hollywood (2018e) *Eligibility for the 'No Animals Were Harmed' Certification*. Available at: http://humanehollywood.org/index.php/component/content/article/11-film-makers/32-eligibility-no-animals-were-harmed (Accessed: 7 September 2018).

Humane Hollywood (2018f) *Pirates of the Caribbean: Cure of the Black Pearl*. Available at: http://humanehollywood.org/index.php/movie-archive/item/pirates-of-the-caribbean-the-curse-of-the-black-pearl (Accessed: 11 September 2018).

Humane Hollywood (2018g) *Snow Buddies*. Available at: http://humanehollywood.org/index.php/movie-archive/item/snow-buddies (Accessed: 8 September 2018).

Humane Hollywood (2019) *Most Frequently Requested Advisories and Guidelines*. Available at: http://humanehollywood.org/index.php/component/content/category/11-film-makers (Accessed: 10 September 2019).

IMDB (2016) *Lady and the Tramp*. Available at: https://www.imdb.com/title/tt0048280/ (Accessed: 22 October 2019).

IMDB (2017) *Bolt*. Available at: https://www.imdb.com/title/tt0397892/ (Accessed: 12 December 2017).

IMDB (2018a) *Andrew Stanton*. Available at: https://www.imdb.com/name/nm0004056/ (Accessed: 9 July 2018).

IMDB (2018b) *Cruella 2020*. Available at: https://www.imdb.com/title/tt3228774/ (Accessed: 22 December 2018).

IMDB (2018c) *Home on the Range*. Available at: https://www.imdb.com/title/tt0299172/releaseinfo (Accessed: 22 November 2018).

IMDB (2018d) *Snow Buddies*. Available at: https://www.imdb.com/title/tt1079448/companycredits?ref_=tt_dt_co (Accessed: 10 September 2018).

IMDB (2019) *101 Dalmatians: The Series*. Available at: https://www.imdb.com/title/tt0144700/ (Accessed: 10 March 2019).

Inge, M. (2004) 'Walt Disney's 'Snow White and the Seven Dwarfs': Art, adaptation and ideology', *Journal Of Popular Film And Television*, 32(3), pp. 132–142.

Jackson, K. M. (1993) *Walt Disney, a Bio-Bibliography*. Westport: Greenwood Press.

Jackson, K. M. (2005) *Walt Disney: Conversations*. Jackson: University Press of Mississippi.

Jeppley, J. (2010) 'Pets and Disney – How Animated Movies Effect the Pet Trade', *That Pet Blog*, 2 September. Available at: http://www.thatpetblog.com/2010/09/02/pets-and-disney-how-animated-movies-effect-the-pet-trade/ (Accessed: 12 October 2018).

Johnson, J. (2002) 'Coonskin Cap Clings to 'Crockett'', *Los Angeles Times*, 23 August. Available at: http://articles.latimes.com/2002/aug/23/local/me-fess23 (Accessed: 12 February 2019).

Johnston, O. and Thomas, F. (1993). *The Disney Villain*. New York: Hyperion Press.

Kalmakurki, M. (2018) 'Snow White and the Seven Dwarfs, Cinderella and Sleeping Beauty: The Components of Costume Design in Disney's Early Hand-Drawn Animated Feature Films', *Animation*, 13(1), pp. 7–19.

Karlson, D. (2013) 'How much is too much for your new favourite coat?', *Glamour*, 8 August. Available at: https://www.glamourmagazine.co.uk/article/cost-of-designer-fashion-fur-coat-more-than-a-house (Accessed: 10 November 2018).

Kassam, A. and Glenza, J. (2015) 'Killer of Cecil the lion was dentist from Minnesota, claim Zimbabwe officials', *The Guardian*, 28 July. Available at: https://www.theguardian.com/environment/2015/jul/28/killer-of-cecil-the-lion-was-american-zimbabwe-officials-claim (Accessed: 5 March 2019).

Kennedy, H. (2018) 'The Myth of the She-Devil: Why we Judge Female Criminals More Harshly', *The Guardian*, 2 October. Available at: https://www.theguardian.com/uk-news/2018/oct/02/the-myth-of-the-she-devil-why-we-judge-female-criminals-more-harshly (Accessed: 23 November 2018).

Khazaal, N. and Almiron, N. (2016) 'An Angry Cow is Not a Good Eating Experience', *Journalism Studies*, 17(3), pp. 374–391.

Kidd, A. H. and Kidd, R. M. (1990) 'Factors in Children's Attitudes Towards Pets', *Psychological Reports*, 66(3), pp. 775–786.

Kipling, R. (1937) *The Works*. London: Macmillan and Company.

Kirk, K. (2013) 'Shopping in Frontierland: A Coonskin Cap', *Walt Disney World for Grown Ups*, 31 July. Available at: http://www.wdwforgrownups.com/articles/shopping-frontierland-coonskin-cap (Accessed: 22 June 2019).

Kogan, L. R. (2013) 'Cats in Animal Shelters: Exploring the Common Perception That Black Cats Take Longer to Adopt', *The Open Veterinary Science Journal*, 7(1), pp. 18–22.

Lamarre, T. (2011) 'Speciesism, Part III: Neoteny and the Politics of Life', *Mechademia*, 6(1), pp. 110–136.

Lancaster, K. and Boyd, J. (2015) 'Redefinition, Differentiation, and the Farm Animal Welfare Debate', *Journal of Applied Communication Research*, 43(2), pp. 185–202.

Langer, M. (1990) 'Regionalism in Disney Animation: Pink Elephants and Dumbo', *Film History*, 4(4), pp. 305–321.

Lawrence, F. (2016) 'If consumers knew how farmed chickens were raised, they might never eat their meat again', *The Guardian*, 24 April. Available at: https://www.theguardian.com/environment/2016/apr/24/real-cost-of-roast-chicken-animal-welfare-farms (Accessed: 22 November 2018).

Layng, J. (2001) 'The Animated Woman: The Powerless Beauty of Disney Heroines from Snow White to Jasmine', *The American Journal of Semiotics*, 17(3), pp. 197–215.

Lazarus, S. (2015) 'Has Sully from Monsters Inc Been Turned into a Toilet Seat Cover?', *Radio Times*, 12 August. Available at: http://www.radiotimes.com/news/2015-08-12/has-sully-from-monsters-inc-been-turned-into-a-toilet-seat-cover/ (Accessed: 24 November 2018).

Leder, D. (2012) 'Old McDonald's Had a Farm: The Metaphysics of Factory Farming', *Journal of Animal Ethics*, 2(1), pp. 73–86.

Leventi-Perez, O. (2011) *Disney's Portrayal of Nonhuman Animals in Animated Films Between 2000 and 2010*. PhD thesis. Georgia State University. Available at: https://scholarworks.gsu.edu/cgi/viewcontent.cgi?article=1084&context=communication_theses (Accessed: 22 December 2018).

Levitt, T. (2018) 'Dairy's 'dirty secret': it's still cheaper to kill male calves than to rear them', *The Guardian*, 26 March. Available at: https://www.theguardian.com/environment/2018/mar/26/dairy-dirty-secret-its-still-cheaper-to-kill-male-calves-than-to-rear-them (Accessed: 17 January 2019).

Loughrey, C. (2017) 'A Dog's Purpose: Terrified Dog Filmed Being Pushed into Water during Shooting', *Independent*, 19 January. Available at: https://www.independent.co.uk/arts-entertainment/films/news/a-dogs-purpose-dog-pushed-into-water-peta-boycott-german-shepherd-a7534741.html (Accessed: 10 January 2019).

Lusher, A. (2003) 'Whale star of 'Free Willy' dies after return to wild', *The Telegraph*, 14 December. Available at: https://www.telegraph.co.uk/news/worldnews/northamerica/usa/1449436/Whale-star-of-Free-Willy-dies-after-return-to-wild.html (Accessed: 14 November 2018).

Lutts, R. H. (1992) 'The Trouble with Bambi: Walt Disney's Bambi and the American Vision of Nature', *Forest & Conservation History*, 36(4), pp. 160–171.

Luz, A. C., Guèze, M., Paneque-Gálvez, J., Pino, J., Macía, M. J., Orta-Martínez, M., and Reyes-García, V. (2015) 'How Does Cultural Change Affect Indigenous Peoples' Hunting Activity? An Empirical Study Among the Tsimane' in the Bolivian Amazon', *Conservation and Society*, 13(4), pp. 382–94.

MacClellan, J. (2013) 'Size Matters: Animal Size, Contributory Causation, and Ethical Vegetarianism', *Journal of Animal Ethics*, 3(1), pp. 57–68.

Mahe, Y. (2011) 'History of Fur in Fashion: Introduction', *Fashion in Time*, 4 December. Available at: http://www.fashionintime.org/history-fur-fashion-introduction/ (Accessed: 22 November 2017).

Marino, L. and Mountain, M. (2015) 'Denial of Death and the Relationship between Humans and Other Animals', *Anthrozoos*, 28(1), pp. 5–21.

McPhedran, S. (2009) 'A Review of the Evidence for Associations between Empathy, Violence, and Animal Cruelty', *Aggression and Violent Behaviour*, 14(1), pp. 1–4.

McRobbie, L. R. (2017) 'Should we stop keeping pets? Why more and more ethicists say yes', *The Guardian*, 1 August. Available at: https://www.theguardian.com/lifeandstyle/2017/aug/01/should-we-stop-keeping-pets-why-more-and-more-ethicists-say-yes (Accessed: 17 December 2018).

McVeigh, T. (2014) 'Animal Rights Campaigners Protest as Fur Comes Back into Fashion', *The Guardian*, 1 March. Available at: https://www.theguardian.com/fashion/2014/mar/01/animal-campaigners-protest-fur-fashion (Accessed: 22 June 2018).

McWilliams, J. (2012) 'PETA's Terrible, Horrible, No Good, Very Bad History of Killing Animals', *The Atlantic*, 12 March. Available at: https://www.theatlantic.com/health/archive/2012/03/petas-terrible-horrible-no-good-very-bad-history-of-killing-animals/254130/ (Accessed: 30 January 2019).

Mechling, J. (2004) 'Picturing Hunting', *Western Folklore*, 63(1/2), pp. 51–78.

Meredith, C. (2013) 'Animals Electrocuted, Strangled and Skinned Alive: The True Face of China's Fur Farms', *Express*, 1 March. Available at: http://www.express.co.uk/news/world/381117/Animals-electrocuted-strangled-and-skinned-alive-The-true-face-of-China-s-fur-farms (Accessed: 16 February 2019).

Mollet, T. (2013) '"With a Smile and a Song...": Walt Disney and the Birth of the American Fairy Tale', *Marvels & Tales*, 27(1), pp. 109–124.

Moore and Giles (2018) *History of Leather*. Available at: https://www.mooreandgiles.com/leather/resources/history/ (Accessed: 2 March 2018).

Mosley, L. (1985) *Disney's World: A Biography*. New York: Stein and Day.

Mosley, M. (2014) 'Can Eating Meat be eco-friendly?', *BBC News*, 20 August. Available at: https://www.bbc.co.uk/news/science-environment-28858289 (Accessed: 27 January 2019).

Mullins, A. (2018) 'URGENT: 'Outdoor Dogs' in Freezing Temps Are Left to Die Slowly and Painfully', *PETA*, 6 December. Available at: https://www.peta.org/blog/urgent-freezing-dogs/ (Accessed: 14 March 2019).

Murguía, S. J. (2018) *The Encyclopedia of Racism in American Films*. Lanham: Rowman & Littlefield Publishers.

National Geographic (2019) *Zoo*. Available at: https://www.nationalgeographic.org/encyclopedia/zoo/ (Accessed: 15 January 2019).

Neff, C. (2015) 'The Jaws Effect: How movie narratives are used to influence policy responses to shark bites in Western Australia', *Australian Journal of Political Science*, 50(1), pp. 114–127.

Nelson, C. and Whitley, D. (2012) *The Idea of Nature in Disney Animation*. Abingdon: Taylor and Francis.

Nelson, F., Kerasote, T., Roger, J., King, H., Bateson, P., Eves, H., Wolf, C., and Yaich, S. (2005) 'The Ethics of Hunting', *Frontiers in Ecology and the Environment*, 3(7), pp. 392–397.

Newkey-Burden, C. (2018) 'Why school trips to abattoirs are essential', *The Guardian*, 3 July. Available at: https://www.theguardian.com/world/shortcuts/2018/jul/03/school-trips-to-abattoirs-essential-countryfile-presenter-tom-heap (Accessed: 7 March 2019).

Newkirk, I. (2009) 'Fish? No, they're 'sea kittens'', *The Guardian*, 14 January. Available at: https://www.theguardian.com/commentisfree/2009/jan/14/fish-overfishing-ethical-peta (Accessed: 14 June 2018).

Newkirk, I. E. (2010) 'Lady Gaga's Meat Dress', *PETA*, 13 September. Available at: https://www.peta.org/blog/lady-gagas-meat-dress/ (Accessed: 19 March 2018).

Nijland, H. et al. (2013) 'Frames and Ambivalence in Context: An Analysis of Hands-On Experts' Perception of the Welfare of Animals in Traveling Circuses in The Netherlands', *Journal of Agricultural and Environmental Ethics*, 26(3), pp. 523–535.

Nobis, N. (2009) 'The "Babe" vegetarians: bioethics, animal minds and moral methodology', in Shapshay S. (ed.) *Bioethics at the movies*. Baltimore: Johns Hopkins University Press, pp. 56–73.

North, R. D. (2000) *Fur and Freedom: In Defence of the Fur Trade*. London: eInstitute of Economic Affairs.

Norwood, F. B. and Lusk, J. (2011) *Compassion, by the Pound: the Economics of Farm Animal Welfare*. Abingdon: Oxford University Press.

O'Connor, J. (2016) 'The Case of the Las Vegas Orangutan Beater Continues to Make History', *PETA*. Available at: https://www.peta.org/blog/case-las-vegas-orangutan-beater-continues-make-history/ (Accessed: 12 January 2019).

O'Connor, T. (2018) 'Why Fashion's Anti-Fur Movement is Winning', *Business of Fashion*, 15 October. Available at: https://www.businessoffashion.com/articles/intelligence/why-fashions-anti-fur-movement-is-winning (Accessed: 5 January 2019).

Olson, K. M. (2013) 'An Epideictic Dimension of Symbolic Violence in Disney's Beauty and the Beast: Inter-generational Lessons in Romanticizing and Tolerating Intimate Partner Violence', *The Quarterly Journal of Speech*, 99(4), pp. 448–480.

One Green Planet (2019) *Amazing Animal Free Circuses*. Available at: https://www.onegreenplanet.org/animalsandnature/amazing-animal-free-circuses/ (Accessed: 6 March 2019).

Orlean, S. (2002) 'Where's Willy?', *The New Yorker*, 15 September. Available at: https://www.newyorker.com/magazine/2002/09/23/wheres-willy (Accessed: 22 March 2019).

Oxford University (2017) *Cecil the Lion's Son Xanda also Shot Dead in Zimbabwe*. Available at: http://www.ox.ac.uk/news/2017-07-21-cecil-lion%E2%80%99s-son-xanda-also-shot-dead-zimbabwe (Accessed: 8 January 2019).

Palgrave Macmillan (2019) *The Palgrave Macmillan Animal Ethics Series*. Available at: https://www.palgrave.com/gp/series/14421 (Accessed: 12 September 2019).

Pallant, C. (2010a) 'Disney-Formalism: Rethinking 'Classic Disney'', *Animation*, 5(3), pp. 341–352.

Pallant, C. (2010b) 'Neo-Disney: Recent Developments in Disney Feature Animation', *New Cinemas: Journal of Contemporary Film*, 8(2), pp. 103–117.

Pallant, C. (2011) *Demystifying Disney: A History of Disney Feature Animation.* London: Continuum.

Parasher, P. (2013) 'Mapping the Imaginary: The Neverland of Disney's Indians', in Cheu, J. (ed.) *Diversity in Disney films: Critical Essays on Race, Ethnicity, Gender, Sexuality and Disability*. Jefferson: McFarland & Company, pp. 38–49.

Payne, K. (2010) 'Why is the death of one million a statistic?', *Psychology Today*, 14 March. Available at: https://www.psychologytoday.com/gb/blog/life-autopilot/201003/why-is-the-death-one-million-statistic (Accessed: 22 January 2019).

Paynter, B. (2014) 'Veal Farmers Adopt More Humane Methods', *The New York Times*, 12 August. Available at: https://www.nytimes.com/2014/08/13/dining/veal-farmers-adopt-more-humane-methods.html (Accessed: 12 November 2018).

Perry, N. and Brandt, P. (2008) 'A Case Study on Cruelty to Farm Animals: Lessons Learned From the Hallmark Meat Packing Case', *Michigan Law Review First Impressions*, 106(1), pp. 117–122.

PETA (2017) *In a Win for Animals, Federal Judge Declares Utah 'Ag-Gag' Law Unconstitutional.* Available at: https://www.peta.org/blog/victory-peta-aldf-challenge-utahs-ag-gag-law/ (Accessed: 4 February 2019).

PETA (2018a) *Animal Shelters.* Available at: https://www.peta.org/issues/animal-companion-issues/animal-shelters/ (Accessed: 22 November 2018).

PETA (2018b) *Experiments on Animals: Overview.* Available at: https://www.peta.org/issues/animals-used-for-experimentation/animals-used-experimentation-factsheets/animal-experiments-overview/ (Accessed: 26 November 2018).

PETA (2018c) *'The Greatest Showman' Cruel Racist History Goes Unmentioned in Flick.* Available at: https://www.peta.org/blog/greatest-showman-cruel-racist-history/ (Accessed: 6 March 2019).

PETA (2019a) *About PETA.* Available at: https://www.peta.org/about-peta/ (Accessed: 29 July 2019).

PETA (2019b) *Animal Actors: Involuntary Performers.* Available at: https://www.peta.org/issues/animals-in-entertainment/animals-used-entertainment-factsheets/animal-actors-command-performances/ (Accessed: 8 January 2019).

PETA (2019c) *Casey Affleck Takes Aim at the Meat Industry in Banned Vegetarian Ad.* Available at: https://www.peta.org/features/casey-affleck-takes-aim-meat-industry-banned-vegetarian-ad/ (Accessed: 7 March 2019).

PETA (2019d) *Circuses*. Available at: https://www.peta.org/issues/animals-in-entertainment/circuses/ (Accessed: 27 July 2019).

PETA (2019e) *Cruel Practices*. Available at: https://www.peta.org/issues/animal-companion-issues/cruel-practices/ (Accessed: 16 March 2019).

PETA (2019f) *Dairy Farm Exposed in Eyewitness Footage*. Available at: https://www.peta.org/videos/dairy-farm-exposed/ (Accessed: 27 January 2019).

PETA (2019g) *Factory Farming: Misery for Animals*. Available at: https://www.peta.org/issues/animals-used-for-food/factory-farming/ (Accessed: 15 September 2019).

PETA (2019h) *Great Apes Used in TV, Film, and Ads*. Available at: https://www.peta.org/features/great-apes-used-tv-movies-ads/ (Accessed: 7 June 2019).

PETA (2019i) *Highway Hellholes: 15 Roadside Zoos on the Blacklist*. Available at: https://www.peta.org/living/entertainment/deadly-destinations/ (Accessed: 12 June 2019).

PETA (2019j) *How to Wear Vegan*. Available at: https://how-to-wear-vegan.peta.org/ (Accessed: 12 January 2019).

PETA (2019k) *Is it Ok to Declaw Cats?* Available at: https://www.peta.org/about-peta/faq/is-it-ok-to-declaw-cats/ (Accessed: 20 March 2019).

PETA (2019l) *Mice and Rats in Laboratories*. Available at: https://www.peta.org/issues/animals-used-for-experimentation/animals-laboratories/mice-rats-laboratories/ (Accessed: 27 July 2019).

PETA (2019m) *Rise of the Planet of the Apes*. Available at: https://www.peta.org/features/rise-planet-apes/ (Accessed: 12 March 2019).

PETA (2019n) *Wool, Fur, and Leather: Hazardous to the Environment*. Available at: https://www.peta.org/issues/animals-used-for-clothing/animals-used-clothing-factsheets/wool-fur-leather-hazardous-environment/ (Accessed: 22 January 2019).

PETA (2019o) *Zoos May Actually Hurt Conservation Efforts, Not Help Them*. Available at: https://www.peta.org/features/zoo-conservation-captive-breeding/ (Accessed: 8 April 2019).

Peterson, M. (2007) 'The Animal Apparatus: From a Theory of Animal Acting to an Ethics of Animal Acts', *The Drama Review*, 51(1), pp. 33–48.

Peterson, M. L. and Farrington, D. P. (2007) 'Cruelty to Animals and Violence to People', *Victims & Offenders*, 2(1), pp. 21–43.

Phillips, K. (2015) 'The ethical evolution of zoos', *ABC Australia*, 21 October. Available at: https://www.abc.net.au/radionational/programs/rearvision/the-ethical-history-of-zoos/6869776 (Accessed: 24 November 2018).

Pierce, J. (2016) *Run, Spot, Run: The Ethics of Keeping Pets*. Chicago: University of Chicago Press.

Pierce, J. and Bekoff, M. (2018) 'A Postzoo Future: Why Welfare Fails Animals in Zoos', *Journal of Applied Animal Welfare Science*, 21(1), pp. 43–48.

Pinto, B. (2004) 'A Retirement Home for Famous Apes', *ABC News*, 31 July. Available at: https://abcnews.go.com/WNT/story?id=131784&page=1 (Accessed: 18 January 2019).

Plumwood, V. (2012) ''Babe': The Tale of the Speaking Meat', in Shannon, L. (ed.) *The Eye of the Crocodile*. Canberra: ANU Press, pp. 55–74.

Polone, G. (2017) 'Gavin Polone on 'A Dog's Purpose' Outcry, What Really Happened and Who is to Blame', *The Hollywood Reporter*, 23 January. Available at: https://www.hollywoodreporter.com/news/gavin-polone-a-dogs-purpose-outcry-what-happened-whos-blame-967160 (Accessed: 18 March 2019).

PR Newswire (2013) 'American Humane Association Responds to The Hollywood Reporter', 25 November. Available at: https://www.prnewswire.com/news-releases/american-humane-association-responds-to-the-hollywood-reporter-233398221.html (Accessed: 16 February 2019).

Preschel, J. (2005) 'Roy Horn Tiger Mauling Case Closed', *CBS News*, 28 June. Available at: https://www.cbsnews.com/news/roy-horn-tiger-mauling-case-closed/ (Accessed: 9 February 2019).

Pringle, H. (1998) 'Neolithic Agriculture: The Slow Birth of Agriculture', *Science*, 282(5393), pp. 1446.

Randhawa, S. (2017) 'Animal rights activists and Inuit clash over Canada's indigenous food traditions', *The Guardian*, 1 November. Available at: https://www.theguardian.com/inequality/2017/nov/01/animal-rights-activists-inuit-clash-canada-indigenous-food-traditions (Accessed: 27 March 2019).

Rees, P. A. (2017) *The Laws Protecting Animals and Ecosystems*. New Jersey: Wiley.

Retired Police Canine Foundation (2019) *Retired Police Canine Foundation*. Available at: http://www.policek9help.com/ (Accessed: 11 January 2019).

Riffel, C. (2012) 'Dissecting Bambi: Multiplanar Photography, the Cel Technique, and the Flowering of Full Animation', *Velvet Light Trap*, 69(1), pp. 3–16.

Roberts, E. (2018) 'Unlocking the Vault', *The Main Street Mouse*, 5 April. Available at: https://www.themainstreetmouse.com/2018/04/05/unlocking-the-vault/ (Accessed: 12 January 2019).

Roderick, K. (1990) 'Spectacle, Complete With Apes, in Vegas Courtroom: Animal rights: Stardust headliner Bobby Berosini is suing after tapes showed him hitting his orang-utans', *LA Times*, 8 August. Available at: https://www.latimes.com/archives/la-xpm-1990-08-08-mn-161-story.html (Accessed: 19 January 2019).

Rose, J. (2010) 'The Fish Feel Little Pain', *NY Times*, 9 August. Available at: https://www.nytimes.com/roomfordebate/2010/08/08/should-fly-fishers-catch-and-always-release/the-fish-feel-little-pain (Accessed: 18 February 2019).

Roth, H. H. (1997) *Wildlife Resources: A Global Account of Economic Use*. New York: Springer.

Rotten Tomatoes (2018) *Earthlings*. Available at: https://www.rottentomatoes.com/m/earthlings_2003/reviews/?page=5&type=user (Accessed 12 November 2018).

Rotten Tomatoes (2019) *Home on the Range*. Available at: https://www.rottentomatoes.com/m/home_on_the_range/ (Accessed: 24 January 2019).

RSPCA (2019a) *Cosmetics Testing Using Animals*. Available at: https://www.rspca.org.uk/adviceandwelfare/laboratory/testingchemicals/cosmetics (Accessed 12 September 2019).

RSPCA (2019b) *Dairy Cows – Farming*. Available at: https://www.rspca.org.uk/adviceandwelfare/farm/dairy/farming (Accessed: 25 April 2019).

Ruston, S. (2007) *Romanticism*. London: Bloomsbury Academic.

Ryder, R. (2004) 'Speciesism revisited', *Think*, 2(6), pp. 83–92.

Safina, C. (2018) 'Are we wrong to assume fish can't feel pain?', *The Guardian*, 30 October. Available at: https://www.theguardian.com/news/2018/oct/30/are-we-wrong-to-assume-fish-cant-feel-pain (Accessed: 18 February 2019).

SAG-AFTRA (2018) *About*. Available at: https://www.sagaftra.org/about (Accessed: 12 September 2018).

Salam, M. (2019) 'What is Toxic Masculinity?', The New York Times, 22 January. Available at: https://www.nytimes.com/2019/01/22/us/toxic-masculinity.html (Accessed: 27 December 2019).

Salten, F. (2013) *Bambi: A Life in the Woods*. New York: Aladdin Paperbacks.

Sanchez, O. (2018) ''Dumbo': Everything to Know About Disney's Live-Action Remake Directed by Tim Burton', *The Hollywood Reporter*, 27 June. Available at: https://www.hollywoodreporter.com/news/dumbo-everything-know-disneys-live-action-remake-1123533 (Accessed: 7 March 2019).

Schatzker, M. (2015) 'Why chicken doesn't taste like chicken anymore', New York Post, 26 April. Available at: https://nypost.com/2015/04/26/why-nothing-especially-chicken-tastes-like-it-used-to/ (Accessed: 12 September 2019).

Scherer, J. (2009) 'Rachel York relishes sharing stage with '101 Dalmatians' Rachel York relishes sharing stage with '101 Dalmatians'', *Boston Herald*, 21 December. Available at: https://www.bostonherald.com/2009/12/21/rachel-york-relishes-sharing-stage-with-101-dalmatians/ (Accessed: 2 February 2018).

Schickel, R. (2019) *The Life, Times, Art, and Commerce of Walt Disney*. New York: Simon and Schuster.

Schlosser, E. (2004) *Fast Food Nation*. New York: Random House.

Schnug, C. (2011) 'The Plight of the Screen Animal: Animal Disappearance and Death on Film', *Film Matters*, 2(2), pp. 18–22.

Scruton, R. (2002) 'Ethics and Welfare: The Case of Hunting', *Philosophy*, 77(302), pp. 543–564.

Sea Shepherd (2019) *Sea Shepherd*. Available at: https://seashepherd.org/ (Accessed: 5 March 2019).

Serpell, J. (1999) 'Working out the beast', in Ascione, F. R. and Arkow P. (eds.) *Child abuse, domestic violence, and animal abuse: Linking the circles of compassion for prevention and intervention*. West Lafayette: Purdue University Press, pp. 38–49.

Serpell, J. (2016) *The Domestic Dog: Its Evolution, Behavior and Interactions with People*. Cambridge: Cambridge University Press.

Sewell, A. (1995) *Black Beauty*. New Edition. London: Penguin Classics.

Shea, M. (2015) 'Punishing Animal Rights Activists for Animal Abuse: Rapid Reporting and the New Wave of Ag-Gag Laws', *Columbia Journal of Law and Social Problems*, 48(3), pp. 337–371.

Sheen, E. (2005) '101 and Counting: Dalmatians in Film and Advertising', *Worldviews: Global Religions, Culture, and Ecology*, 9(2), pp. 236–254.

Shoard, C. (2017) 'A Dog's Purpose Premiere Cancelled After Video of Stunt Dog 'in Distress'', *The Guardian*, 20 January. Available at: https://www.theguardian.com/film/2017/jan/20/a-dogs-purpose-premiere-video-german-shepherd (Accessed: 18 February 2019).

Shop Disney (2019a) *Bambi*. Available at: https://www.shopdisney.co.uk/disney/movies/bambi (Accessed: 10 July 2019).

Shop Disney (2019b) *Characters*. Available at: https://www.shopdisney.co.uk/characters (Accessed: 12 April 2019).

Shop Disney (2019c) *Cruella De Vil*. Available at: https://www.shopdisney.com/characters/cruella-de-vil (Accessed: 16 March 2019).

Shop Disney (2019d) *Fur*. Available at: https://www.shopdisney.com/search?query=fur (Accessed: 27 July 2019).

Shop Disney (2019e) *Lady and the Tramp*. Available at: https://www.shopdisney.co.uk/search?q=lady+tramp (Accessed: 27 July 2019).

Shop Disney (2019f) *Leather Bracelet*. Available at: https://www.shopdisney.com/search?query=leather%20bracelet (Accessed: 18 March 2019).

Shuttlewood, C. Z., Greenwell, P. J., and Montrose, V. T. (2016) 'Pet Ownership, Attitude Toward Pets, and Support for Wildlife Management Strategies', *Human Dimensions of Wildlife*, 21(2), pp. 180–188.

Siegle, L. (2016) 'Is it time to give up leather?', *The Guardian*, 13 March. Available at: https://www.theguardian.com/fashion/2016/mar/13/is-it-time-to-give-up-leather-animal-welfare-ethical-lucy-siegle (Accessed: 25 March 2019).

Simon, S. (2009) 'Indigenous Peoples and Hunting Rights', in Mendes, E. P. and Srighanthan, S. (eds.) *Confronting Discrimination and Inequality in China: Chinese and Canadian Perspectives*. Ottawa: University of Ottawa Press, pp. 405–421.

Simpson, J. (2001) *Foundations of Fiction*. iUniverse.

Singer, G. (2004) 'Home Sweet Home', *Animation World Network*, 2 April. Available at: https://www.awn.com/animationworld/home-sweet-home (Accessed: 16 March 2019).

Singer, P. (1975). *Animal liberation*. New York: Random House.

Singer, P. (1990). *Animal liberation*. 2nd edition. New York: Avon Books.

Singer, P. (1995) *Rethinking Life & Death: The Collapse of Our Traditional Ethics*. Oxford: Oxford UP.

Singer, P. (2009) *Animal Liberation*. Updated Edition. New York: Harper Perennial.

Singer, P. (2015a) *Animal Liberation*. New edition with an introduction by Yuval Noah Harari. London: The Bodley Head.

Singer, P. (2015b) 'The abuse of animals won't stop until we stop eating meat', *The Guardian*, 11 February. Available at: https://www.theguardian.com/commentisfree/2015/feb/11/abuse-animals-meat-eating-industry-liberation-speciesism (Accessed: 14 April 2019).

Sinmez, C. C., Yigit, A., and Aslim, G. (2017) 'Tail docking and ear cropping in dogs: a short review of laws and welfare aspects in the Europe and Turkey', *Italian Journal of Animal Science*, 16(3), pp. 431–437.

Sladen, S. (2015) 'The death of the Dame? Tales from the National Database of Pantomime Performance', *Studies in Theatre and Performance*, 35(1), pp, 80–89.

Smith, D. (1967) *The Starlight Barking*. London: Egmont UK

Smith, D. (2010) *The Hundred and One Dalmatians*. London: Egmont UK.

Smith, D. and Clark, S. (2002) *Disney: The First 100 Years*. Glendale: Disney Publishing.

Snetiker, M. (2014) "Descendants': Meet the evil kids of Disney villains', *Entertainment Weekly*, 16 June. Available at: https://ew.com/article/2014/06/16/disney-descendants/ (Accessed: 14 December 2018).

SPANA (2019a) *Then and Now*. Available at: https://spana.org/thenandnow/ (Accessed: 4 April 2019).

SPANA (2019b) *What are Working Horses?* Available at: https://spana.org/blog/what-are-working-horses/ (Accessed: 4 April 2019).

Spector, A. J. (1998) 'Disney Does Diversity: The Social Context of Racial-Ethnic Imagery', in Kamalipour, Y. R. and Carilli T. (eds.) *Cultural Diversity and the U.S. Media*. New York: State University of New York Press.

Spencer, S., Decuypere, E., Aerts, S., and Tavernier, J. (2006) 'History and Ethics of Keeping Pets: Comparison with Farm Animals', in *Journal of Agricultural and Environmental Ethics*, 19(1), pp. 17–25.

Stafford, E. (2017) 'Hercules' Choice: Virtue, Vice and the Hero of the Twentieth Century Screen', in Almagor, E. and Maurice, L. (eds.) *The Reception of Ancient Virtues and Vices in Modern Popular Culture: Beauty, Bravery, Blood and Glory*. Leiden: Brill.

Stanton, R. R. (2017) 'Speak of the Devil! The Keys to Cruella's Success', *Animation Studies*, 12 June. Available at: https://blog.animationstudies.org/?p=2049 (Accessed: 22 June 2019).

Stanton, R. R. (2019) 'Dark Horse: An Overview of Walt Disney Animation Studios' Horses', *Animation Studies*, 6 May. Available at: https://blog.animationstudies.org/?p=3063 (Accessed: 19 June 2019).

Starkey, P. (2000) 'The history of working animals in Africa', in Blench, R. M. and MacDonald, K. (eds.) *The origins and development of African livestock: archaeology, genetics, linguistics and ethnography*. London: University College London Press, pp. 478–502.

Stevens, P. M. C. and McAlister, E. (2007) 'Ethics in Zoos', *International Zoo Yearbook*, 38(1), pp. 94–101.

Stewart, K. and Cole, M. (2009) 'The Conceptual Separation of Food and Animals', *Childhood, Food, Culture & Society*, 12(4), pp. 457–476.

Stoddart, H. (2004) 'Animals in Sport and Entertainment', *The Reference Librarian*, 41(86), pp. 25–36.

Stokes, J. (2004) 'Lion Griefs: the Wild Animal Act as Theatre', *New Theatre Quarterly*, 20(2), pp. 138–154.

Strodder, C. (2015) *The Disneyland Book of Lists*. Santa Monica: Santa Monica Press.

Sullivan, D. H. (2012) *Our Canine Companions*. Kindle Edition.

Sullivan, K. (2017) 'I finally watched 'Earthlings' and wow, was I unprepared', *PETA*, 11 May. Available at: https://www.peta.org/features/i-finally-watched-earthlings/ (Accessed: 17 March 2019).

Surendra, P. (2019) 'The Grand National: 9 things they don't tell you about horse racing', *PETA*, 2 April. Available at: https://www.peta.org.uk/blog/the-grand-national-9-things-they-dont-tell-you-about-horse-racing/ (Accessed: 26 June 2019).

Teurlay, F. (2014) 'Recap: Lady and the Tramp – A Technical Triumph', *Walt Disney*, 28 May. Available at: https://www.waltdisney.org/blog/recap-lady-and-tramp-technical-triumph (Accessed: 16 January 2019).

The Daily Telegraph (2009) PETA's latest idiotic demand – fish are 'sea kittens'. Available at: https://www.dailytelegraph.com.au/petas-latest-idiotic-demand-fish-are-sea-kittens/news-story/1d2aa0676c0336dbe223fdc4e75576e3?sv=e486ff3785a3216232146c7cc809add9 (Accessed: 22 January 2019).

The Ecologist (2009) *Hell for Leather*. Available at: https://www.youtube.com/watch?v=4A6siB9B4Ak (Accessed: 12 February 2019).

The Guardian (2008) *Don't Hide From the Truth*, 27 August. Available at: https://www.theguardian.com/lifeandstyle/2008/aug/27/ethicalfashion.leather (Accessed: 17 January 2018).

The Guardian (2017) *'Greatest show on Earth': Ringling Bros circus bows out after 146 years*, 22 May. Available at: https://www.theguardian.com/stage/2017/may/22/ringling-bros-barnum-bailey-circus-final-show-new-york-146-years (Accessed: 23 December 2018).

The Guardian (2018), *Deer poacher ordered to watch Bambi once a month in jail*, 18 December. Available at: https://www.theguardian.com/us-news/2018/dec/18/deer-poacher-ordered-to-watch-bambi-once-a-month-in-jail (Accessed: 27 December 2018).

The Jane Goodall Institute Australia (2018) *Great Apes*. Available at: https://www.janegoodall.org.au/great-apes/ (Accessed: 8 September 2018).

The Kennel Club (2019a) *Novice Breeder Checklist*. Available at: https://www.thekennelclub.org.uk/breeding/breeding-from-your-dog/novice-breeder-checklist/ (Accessed: 8 July 2019).

The Kennel Club (2019b) *Where not to buy a dog: puppy farms, puppy dealers and pet shops*. Available at: https://www.thekennelclub.org.uk/getting-a-dog-or-puppy/finding-the-right-breeder/where-not-to-buy-a-dog/ (Accessed: 8 July 2019).

The Numbers (2019a) *101 Dalmatians (1996)*. Available at: https://www.the-numbers.com/movie/101-Dalmatians-(1996)#tab=summary (Accessed: 4 July 2019).

The Numbers (2019b) *Home on the Range (2004)*. Available at: https://www.the-numbers.com/movie/Home-on-the-Range#tab=summary (Accessed: 22 March 2019).

The Numbers (2019) *Lady and the Tramp (1955)*. Available at: https://www.the-numbers.com/movie/Lady-and-the-Tramp#tab=summary (Accessed: 19 January 2019).

The Numbers (2019d) *Snow Buddies (2008)*. Available at: https://www.the-numbers.com/movie/Snow-Buddies#tab=summary (Accessed: 15 March 2019).

The Official Disney Fan Club (2018) *Disney's Decades of Work with American Humane Association*. Available at: https://d23.com/disney-aha-historic-milestones/ (Accessed: 18 September 2018).

The Telegraph (2002) *Dressage chiefs forced to combat 'unacceptable' cruelty*, 12 May. Available at: https://www.telegraph.co.uk/news/uknews/1393943/Dressage-chiefs-forced-to-combat-unacceptable-cruelty.html (Accessed: 16 March 2019).

The Telegraph (2017) *A movie Easter Egg hunt: the best hidden messages and inside jokes in film*, 17 April. Available at: https://www.telegraph.co.uk/films/0/movie-easter-eggs-hunt-best-hidden-messages-inside-jokes-film/lion-kings-scar-makes-morbid-cameo-hercules/ (Accessed: 7 March 2019).

The Vegan Society (2019) *Statistics*. Available at: https://www.vegansociety.com/news/media/statistics (Accessed: 1 July 2019).

The Walt Disney Family Museum (2011) *The Timely "Dumbo": Almost a Cover Boy*. Available at: https://www.waltdisney.org/blog/timely-dumbo-almost-cover-boy (Accessed: 28 March 2018).

Thomas, B. (1976) *Walt Disney: An American Original*. New York: Simon & Schuster.

Thomas, B. (1994) *Walt Disney: An American Original*. Glendale: Disney Publishing Worldwide.

Thomas, B. (1998) *Building a Company: Roy O. Disney and the Creation of an Entertainment Empire*. Glendale: Disney Publishing.

Thomas, F. and Johnston, O. (1981) *Disney Animation: The Illusion of Life*. Glendale: Disney Publishing Worldwide.

Tiplady, C. et al. (2013) 'Public Response to Media Coverage of Animal Cruelty', *Journal of Agricultural and Environmental Ethics*, 26(4), pp. 869–885.

Tobias, R. (2011) *Film and the American Moral Vision of Nature: Theodore Roosevelt to Walt Disney*. East Lansing: Michigan State University Press.

Tonsor, G. T. and Widmar, N. J. O. (2012) 'Impacts of Animal Well-being and Welfare Media on Meat Demand', *Journal of Agricultural Economics*, 62(1), pp. 59–72.

Urquhart, S. (1991) 'What Becomes a Legend Least?', *Time*, 19 August. Available at: http://content.time.com/time/magazine/article/0,9171,973656,00.html (Accessed: 11 November 2018).

Valkenburg, P. M. (2004) *Children's Responses to the Screen A Media Psychological Approach*. Hoboken: Taylor and Francis.

Van der Zee, B. (2018) 'What is the true cost of eating meat?', *The Guardian*, 7 May. Available at: https://www.theguardian.com/news/2018/may/07/true-cost-of-eating-meat-environment-health-animal-welfare (Accessed: 28 November 2018).

Vandersommers, D. (2017) 'What's All Happening at the Zoo?', *Origins*, 10(6). Available at: https://origins.osu.edu/article/whats-all-happening-zoo (Accessed: 6 December 2018).

Vegan Life Magazine (2017) *The 'Leftover' Leather Lie Exposed*, 10 October. Available at: https://www.veganlifemag.com/leather-lie-exposed/ (Accessed: 12 November 2018).

Vonledebur, C. (2013) 'Leamington Game of Thrones actress Sophie Turner enjoying her rise to fame', *Coventry Telegraph*, 16 August. Available at: https://www.coventrytelegraph.net/whats-on/film-tv/leamington-game-thrones-actress-sophie-5740234 (Accessed: 3 December 2018).

Wadewitz, L. (2011) 'Are Fish Wildlife?', *Environmental History*, 16(3), pp. 423–427.

Walker, J. P. (2015) *The Legendary Mountain Men of North America*. Morrisville: Lulu Books.

Wasko, J. (2001) *Understanding Disney: The Manufacture of Fantasy*. Cambridge: Polity Press.

Wasley, A., Harvey, F., Davies, M., and Child, D. (2017) 'UK has nearly 800 livestock mega farms, investigation reveals', *The Guardian*, 19 June. Available at: https://www.theguardian.com/environment/2017/jul/17/uk-has-nearly-800-livestock-mega-farms-investigation-reveals (Accessed: 22 October 2018).

Wasley, A., Cook, C. D., and Jones, N. (2018) 'Two Amputations a Week: The Cost of Working in a US meat plant', *The Guardian*, 5 July. Available at: https://www.theguardian.com/environment/2018/jul/05/amputations-serious-injuries-us-meat-industry-plant (Accessed: 12 February 2019).

Watson, K. W. (2015) "Dolphin Safe' Labels On Canned Tuna Are A Fraud', *Forbes*, 29 April. Available at: https://www.forbes.com/sites/real-spin/2015/04/29/dolphin-safe-labels-on-canned-tuna-are-a-fraud/#699a602c295e (Accessed: 2 December 2018).

Watts, S. (1995) 'Walt Disney: Art and Politics in the American Century', *The Journal of American History*, 82(1), pp. 84–110.

Weaver, M. and Gajanan, M. (2015) 'Cecil the lion hunter Walter Palmer faces calls for prosecution', *The Guardian*, 29 July. Available at: https://www.theguardian.com/world/2015/jul/29/cecil-the-lion-calls-for-prosecution-us-dentist-walter-palmer (Accessed: 12 September 2019).

Webb, S. (2015) 'The Russian restaurant where LEOPARD and TIGER meat is on the menu', *Mirror*, 27 July. Available at: https://www.mirror.co.uk/news/world-news/russian-restaurant-leopard-tiger-meat-5109233 (Accessed: 12 September 2019).

Weisberger, M. (2017) 'Hunting Big Game: Why People Kill Animals for Fun', *Scientific American*, 28 May. Available at: https://www.scientificamerican.com/article/hunting-big-game-why-people-kill-animals-for-fun/ (Accessed: 19 February 2019).

Wells, P. (1998) *Understanding Animation*. London: Routledge.

Wells, P. (2008) *The Animated Bestiary: Animals, Cartoons, and Culture*. New Brunswick: Rutgers University Press.

Wells, P. (2013) 'Thou Art Translated' Analysing Animated Adaptation', in Cartmell, D. and Whelehan, I. (eds.) *Adaptations: From Text to Screen, Screen to Text*. Florence: Taylor and Francis, pp. 199–213.

Westbury, H. R. and Neumann, D. L. (2008) 'Empathy-related Responses to Movie Film Stimuli Depicting Human and Non-Human Animal Targets in Negative Circumstances', *Biological Psychology*, 78(1), pp. 66–74.

Whitley, D. (2008) *The Idea of Nature in Disney Animation*. Routledge: London.

Willis, K. and Ludlow, R. (2015) *Raising Chickens For Dummies*. Hoboken: John Wiley & Sons.

Wills, J. (2014) 'Nature writes the screenplays': Felix Salten and Disney Nature in Bambi (1942), Perri (1957) and The Shaggy Dog (1959)', in Jackson, K. M. and West, M. I. (eds.) *Walt Disney and His Narratives: From Reader to Storyteller*. Jefferson: McFarland & Co., pp. 45–61.

Wills, J. (2017) *Disney Culture*. New Jersey: Rutgers University Press.

Wills, S. (2012) 'The Crowded, Competitive World of Animal Acting', *The Atlantic*, 31 May. Available at: https://www.theatlantic.com/entertainment/archive/2012/05/the-crowded-competitive-world-of-animal-acting/257897/ (Accessed: 21 September 2019).

Wilson, D. A. H. (2017) 'Circus animals and the illusion of wildness', *Early Popular Visual Culture*, 15(3), pp. 350–366.

World Population Review (2019) *World Population 2019*. Available at: http://worldpopulationreview.com/continents/world-population/ (Accessed: 22 January 2019).

Wrenn, C. L. (2017) 'Skeptics and 'The White Stuff': Promotion of Cows' Milk and Other Nonhuman Animal Products in the Skeptic Community as Normative Whiteness', *Relations. Beyond Anthropocentrism*, 5(1), pp. 72–81.

Yeginsu, C. (2018) 'Croydon Cat Killer: London Police Solve a Mystery', *The New York Times*, 20 September. Available at: https://www.nytimes.com/2018/09/20/world/europe/london-cat-killer.html (Accessed: 5 June 2019).

Yount, L. (2008) *Animal Rights*. New York: Infobase.

Youtube (2019) *PETA (People for the Ethical Treatment of Animals)*. Available at: https://www.youtube.com/channel/UCmQRypK6kAcujJAlYZpFW8Q (Accessed: 13 June 2019).

Yuhas, A. (2015) 'A third of Americans believe animals deserve same rights as people, poll finds', *The Guardian*, 19 May. Available at: https://www.theguardian.com/world/2015/may/19/americans-animals-human-rights-poll (Accessed: 22 May 2019).

Zampa, M. (2019) 'How Many Animals Are Killed for Food Every Day?', *Sentient Media*. Available at: https://sentientmedia.org/how-many-animals-are-killed-for-food-every-day/ (Accessed: 12 March 2019).

Zawistowski, S. and Reid, P. (2016) 'Dogs in today's society: The role of applied animal behaviour', in J. Serpell (ed.) *The Domestic Dog: Its Evolution, Behavior and Interactions with People*. Cambridge: Cambridge University Press, pp. 227–244.

Zencey, E. (1987) 'On Hunting', *The North American Review*, 272(2), pp. 59–63.

Films

101 Dalmatians (1996) Directed by Herek, S. [Film]. California: Buena Vista Pictures Distribution.

101 Dalmatians II: Patch's London Adventure (2003) Directed by Kammerud J. and Smith, B. [Film]. California: Disney Television Animation.

A Dogs Purpose (2017) Directed by Hallström, L. [Film]. Glendale: DreamWorks et al.

Aladdin (1992) Directed by Clements, R. and Musker, J. [Film]. California: Walt Disney Productions.

Alice in Wonderland (1951) Directed by Geronimi C. et al. [Film]. California: Walt Disney Productions.

Atlantis: The Lost Empire (2001) Directed by Trousdale, G. and Wise, K. [Film]. California: Walt Disney Productions.

Babe (1995) Directed by Noonan, C. [Film]. California: Universal Pictures.

Bambi (1942) Directed by Algar, J. et al. [Film]. California: Walt Disney Productions.

Beauty and the Beast (1991) Directed by Trousdale, G. and Wise, K. [Film]. California: Walt Disney Productions.

Big Hero 6 (2014) Directed by Hall, D. and Williams, C. [Film]. California: Walt Disney Productions.

Bolt (2008) Directed by Williams, C. and Howard, B. [Film]. California: Walt Disney Productions.

Brother Bear (2003) Directed by Blaise, A. and Walker, R. [Film]. California: Walt Disney Productions.

Chicken Little (2005) Directed by Dindal, M. [Film]. California: Walt Disney Productions.

Chicken Run (2000) Directed by Lord, P. and Park, N. [Film]. California: DreamWorks Pictures.

Cinderella (1950) Directed by Geronimi, C. et al. [Film]. California: Walt Disney Productions.

Descendants (2015) Directed by Ortega, K. [Film]. California: Disney – ABC Domestic Television.

Dinosaur (2000) Directed by Zondag, R. and Leighton, E. [Film]. California: Walt Disney Productions.

Dominion (2018) Directed by Delforce, C. [Film]. Available at: https://www.dominionmovement.com/ (Accessed: 22 June 2019).

Dumbo (1941) Directed by Armstrong, S. et al. [Film]. California: Walt Disney Productions.

Dumbo (2019) Directed by Burton, T. [Film]. California: Walt Disney Studios Motion Pictures.

Earthlings (2005) Directed by Monson, S. [Film]. Nation Earth.

Fantasia (1940) Directed by Algar J. et al. [Film]. California: Walt Disney Productions.

Fantasia 2000 (1999) Directed by Hahn, D. et al. [Film]. California: Walt Disney Productions.

Free Willy (1993) Directed by Wincer, S. [Film]. California: Warner Bros.

Frozen (2013) Directed by Buck, C. and Lee, J. [Film]. California: Walt Disney Productions.

Fun and Fancy Free (1947) Directed by Geronimi, C. et al. [Film]. California: Walt Disney Productions.

Hercules (1997) Directed by Clements R. & Musker J. [Film]. California: Walt Disney Productions.

Home on the Range (2004) Directed by Finn, W. and Sanford, J. [Film]. California: Walt Disney Productions.

Jaws (1975) Directed by Spielberg, S. [Film]. California: Universal Pictures.

Lady and the Tramp (1955) Directed by Geronimi, C. et al. [Film]. California: Walt Disney Productions.

Life of Pi (2012) Directed by Lee, A. [Film]. California: 20th Century Fox.

Lilo & Stitch (2002) Directed by Sanders, C. and DeBlois, D. [Film]. California: Walt Disney Productions.

Make Mine Music (1946) Directed by Cormack, R. et al. [Film]. California: Walt Disney Productions.

Meet the Robinsons (2007) Directed by Anderson, S. J. [Film]. California: Walt Disney Productions.

Melody Time (1948) Directed by Scribner, G. [Film]. California: Walt Disney Productions.

Moana (2016) Directed by Clements, R. and Murker, J. [Film]. California: Walt Disney Productions.

Monsters, Inc. (2001) Directed by Docter, P. [Film]. California: Walt Disney Pictures.

Mulan (1998) Directed by Cook, B. and Bancroft, T. [Film]. California: Walt Disney Productions.

Oliver & Company (1988) Directed by Lounsbery J. et al. [Film]. California: Walt Disney Productions.

One Hundred and One Dalmatians (1961) Directed by Geronimi, C. et al. [Film]. California: Walt Disney Productions.

Partysaurus Rex (2012) Directed by Walsh, M. [Film]. California: Walt Disney Studios Motion Pictures.

Peter Pan (1953) Directed by Geronimi C. et al. [Film]. California: Walt Disney Productions.

Pinocchio (1940) Directed by Ferguson, N. et al. [Film]. California: Walt Disney Productions.

Pocahontas (1995) Directed by Gabriel, M. and Goldberg, E. [Film]. California: Walt Disney Productions.

Ratatouille (2007) Bird, B. [Film]. California: Walt Disney Studios Motion Picture.

Robin Hood (1973) Directed by Reitherman, W. et al. [Film]. California: Walt Disney Productions.

Saludos Amigos (1942) Directed by Jackson, W. et al. [Film]. California: Walt Disney Productions.

Schindler's List (1993) Directed by Spielberg, S. [Film] California: Universal Pictures.

Sleeping Beauty (1959) Directed by Geronimi, C. et al. [Film]. California: Walt Disney Productions.

Snow White and the Seven Dwarfs (1937) Directed by Cottrell, W. et al. [Film] California: Walt Disney Productions.

Tangled (2010) Directed by Greno, N. and Howard, B. [Film]. California: Walt Disney Productions.

Tarzan (1999) Directed by Buck, C. and Lima, K. [Film]. California: Walt Disney Productions.

The Adventures of Ichabod and Mr. Toad (1949) Directed by Algar, J. et al. [Film]. California: Walt Disney Productions.

The Aristocats (1970) Directed by Reitherman, W. et al. [Film]. California: Walt Disney Productions.

The Artist (2011) Directed by Hazanavicius, M. [Film]. France: Warner Bros.

The Black Cauldron (1985) Directed by Berman, T. et al. [Film]. California: Walt Disney Productions.

The Emperor's New Groove (2000) Directed by Dindal, M. [Film]. California: Walt Disney Productions.

The Fox and the Hound (1981) Directed by Stevens, A. et al. [Film]. California: Walt Disney Productions.

The Great Mouse Detective (1986) Directed by Clements, R. et al. [Film]. California: Walt Disney Productions.

The Hunchback of Notre Dame (1996) Directed by Trousdale, G. and Wise, K. [Film]. California: Walt Disney Productions.

The Jungle Book (1967) Directed by Reitherman, W. et al. [Film]. California: Walt Disney Productions.

The Lion King (1994) Directed by Allers, R. and Minkoff, R. [Film]. California: Walt Disney Productions.

The Little Mermaid (1989) Directed by Clements, R. and Musker, J. [Film]. California: Walt Disney Productions.

The Many Adventures of Winnie the Pooh (1977) Directed by Lounsbery J. et al. [Film]. California: Walt Disney Productions.

The Princess and the Frog (2009) Directed by Clements, R. and Musker, J. [Film]. California: Walt Disney Productions.
The Rescuers (1977) Directed by Lounsbery J. et al. [Film]. California: Walt Disney Productions.
The Rescuers Down Under (1990) Directed by Butoy, H. and Gabriel, M. [Film]. California: Walt Disney Productions.
The Sword in the Stone (1963) Directed by Reitherman, W. et al. [Film]. California: Walt Disney Productions.
The Texas Chain Saw Massacre (1974) Directed by Hooper, T. [Film]. United States: Vortex.
The Three Caballeros (1944) Directed by Ferguson, N. et al. [Film]. California: Walt Disney Productions.
Treasure Planet (2002) Directed by Clements, R. and Musker, J. [Film]. California: Walt Disney Productions.
Watership Down (1978) Directed by Rosen, M. [Film]. London: Cinema International Corporation.
We Bought a Zoo (2011) Directed by Crowe, C. [Film]. California: 20th Century Fox.
White Wilderness (1958) Directed by Algar, J. [Film]. California: Buena Vista.
Winnie the Pooh (2011) Directed by Anderson, S. J. and Hall, D. [Film]. California: Walt Disney Productions.
Wreck-It Ralph (2012) Directed by Moore, R. [Film]. California: Walt Disney Productions.
Zootopia (2016) Directed by Howard, B. and Moore, R. [Film]. California: Walt Disney Productions.

Index[1]

[1] Note: Page numbers followed by 'n' refer to notes.

R. Stanton, *The Disneyfication of Animals*, The Palgrave Macmillan Animal Ethics Series, https://doi.org/10.1007/978-3-030-49316-5

The manufacturer's authorised representative in the EU is Springer
Nature Customer Service Centre GmbH, Europaplatz 3, 69115 Heidelberg,
Germany. If you have any concerns regarding our products, please
contact ProductSafety@springernature.com

Printed and bound by CPI Group (UK) Ltd, Croydon, CR0 4YY
30/09/2026
02225645-0003